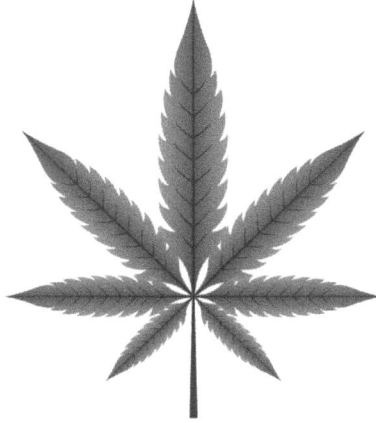

GANJA

*The Virgin Drug
with a Wild Side–It's Good, Bad,
Evil, and Amazing!*

By
Innocent Karikoga

This publication provides content related to educational, medical, and psychological topics; however, it is not intended to be a substitute for the medical advice of a licensed physician. The the reader should consult with their doctor on any matters relating to his/her health. All matters regarding health require medical supervision. It is the responsibility of the reader to comply with their current and future medical treatments and advice.

Further, understand that the guidance contained herein is not intended as a substitute for consultation with a licensed medical, educational, or health care professional and usage of the material implies the acceptance of this disclaimer. Before beginning any change in lifestyle in any way, it is recommended to consult a licensed professional to ensure that one is doing what is best for one's own situation.

The intent of this book is to enlighten readers with a simplified and basic understanding of cannabis and the way it affects our bodies in a general sense. The information found in this book is refined excerpts from the most recent editions of some of the most comprehensive medical textbooks. No claims without scientific explanations are found in this book.

Second Edition.

ISBN: 978-1-9994359-7-4

Contents

- The Three Standard Methods Of Cannabis Consumption
- From Your Breath To Your Circulatory System
- What is cannabis?
- What happens when cannabis enters your brain?
- What causes the variations in cannabis effects in different people?
- What is respiration?
- Oxygen's Journey After Leaving Your Lungs
- What Is Dalton's Law Of Partial Pressure?
- What Happens When Partial Pressures Are Disturbed?
- How Do Your Alveoli Participate In Respiration?
- How Do Your Capillaries Participate In Respiration?
- How Does Cannabis Affect Normal Gas Exchange?
- What Is Hypoxia?

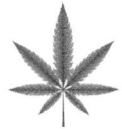

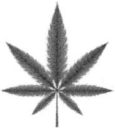

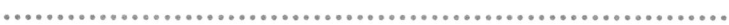

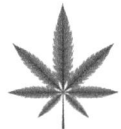

7

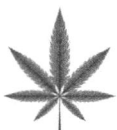

8

- Psychological dependence
- Social dependence
- Cannabis Dependence

- The Basics of Cannabis Metabolism
- The effect of frequent consumption
- Cannabis and Enzyme Induction
- The Effect of Alcohol on OCPs
- The Importance of Your Liver in Drug Metabolism
- The Metabolism of Alcohol
- Alcohol tolerance and interaction with other drugs
- Cannabis Liver Metabolism
- Liver Enzymes and Drug Inhibition
- Example of Drug Interaction
- Cannabis and Drug Interaction
- Enzyme Variations Among Different Populations
- The Effect of Muscle and Fat on cannabis distribution
- Effect of Hormonal Difference on Cannabis Efficacy
- Chronic Cannabis Use, Storage, Release from Storage, and Testing
- Some Social Challenges and Complications of Cannabis Use

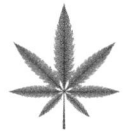

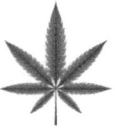

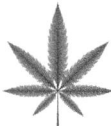

11

Preface

In a fascinating world where scientific objectivity has been thrown out the window, it's genuinely remarkable how those lacking education and knowledge in socially controversial fields manage to rise to the top. All it takes is a loud voice, and voila! You're suddenly leading society in a bold new direction. Forget about being informed or educated on a topic because now it's all about who can shout the loudest in a conversation or debate.

As a delightful consequence, the masses gravitate towards repeated false claims, not because they have any merit whatsoever but simply because these claims have been screamed into their ears so often that any opposition has thrown in the towel. Who needs facts and evidence when you can drown out reason with sheer volume?

Of course, when dealing with matters of metaphysical interest, it's easy to pay no heed to this tidal wave of disinformation. After all, the repercussions of such cult-like arguments are practically negligible in the grand scheme. But when false statements, misconceptions, and misconstrued statements can have deadly long-term physical and psychological consequences, it becomes imperative to oppose these unsubstantiated claims vehemently.

And that brings us to the delightful world of cannabis. Brace yourself because we're about to embark on a riveting exploration of this plant, from its very essence to its impact on the population. But hold your horses! Before we start freely handing out cannabis to anyone who asks for it, it might be wise to gain an objective understanding first.

We've all heard the saying, "You can have your own opinions, but you can't have your own facts." Well, even within the realm of freedom of speech, we should be wary of dire consequences. Sure, cannabis might be a

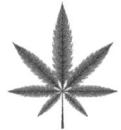

13

hoot to consume, but let's not forget that some individuals suffer from its physical and mental adverse effects. While some folks argue for the benefits of cannabis, and they're not entirely wrong, we must weigh the risks and benefits on both personal and population levels.

Suppose you're seeking validation for your strong opinions on cannabis. In that case, whether they're wildly positive or negative, you should reconsider your choice of reading material. This book demands an open mind, a willingness to learn, and a healthy dose of humility to acknowledge that your long-held and fiercely defended views on cannabis may be objectively wrong.

Some think cannabis is a godsend, while others are convinced it's the devil's lettuce. And let's not forget the folks who fall somewhere in between, finding it both marvellous and dreadful. They might all be right, or they might all be wrong. But we may never truly know without delving into the subject matter and exploring the objective knowledge behind the drug.

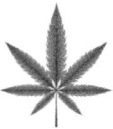

14

So, my dear readers, let's buckle up and dive headfirst into the thrilling world of cannabis. It's bound to be an enlightening adventure where we challenge our preconceived notions and embrace the possibility that we might have been barking up the wrong tree all along. Let the journey begin!

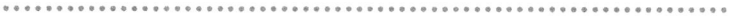

Introduction

Prepare yourself for a riveting expedition into the realm of cannabis, where we shall embark on a quest to unravel the mysteries surrounding its benefits and effects. Our mission? To arm you with knowledge and approach this topic objectively, enabling you to make well-informed decisions.

Now, I must warn you, this journey isn't for the faint of heart. Cannabis, you see, has garnered a reputation as a harmful substance with addictive properties and a range of adverse health consequences. For some, this's reason enough to make it illegal forever. Others argue for its decriminalization but hesitate to fully legalize it, fearing that such a move would send the wrong message to impressionable young minds. It's a debate that wobbles back and forth like a delicate balancing act.

This topic is a hotbed of contention. On one side, some champion the potential benefits of cannabis, while on the other, a camp staunchly warns of its dangers. To arrive at a well-rounded understanding, we must consider both perspectives, carefully examining the evidence presented.

15

In science, falsehoods don't magically transform into truths, and erroneous beliefs don't suddenly become right. Evil doesn't become acceptable simply because the majority embraces it. Science, you see, operates on a different plane altogether, devoid of the democratic principles that govern other aspects of society. It's not uncommon for the majority to be proven wrong by the lone voice of an objective scientist, shattering their preconceived notions in a single revelatory moment.

The push against the boundaries of conventional wisdom, and the defiance of the majority mindset, has often been the catalyst for groundbreaking discoveries and scientific advancements. So, my brave companions, let's not be swayed by the tide of popular opinion alone.

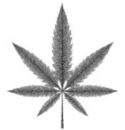

Instead, let's embrace the spirit of intellectual curiosity and critical thinking as we venture forth into the realm of cannabis.

Remember, the quest for knowledge requires an open mind, a willingness to question established beliefs, and the courage to accept that someone with superior intelligence may shatter our preconceptions. Together, we shall navigate the complex tapestry of cannabis, unravel its intricacies, and emerge on the other side equipped with the wisdom necessary to navigate this captivating domain.

Ganja-the virgin drug with a wild side: was written from a medical perspective. With a scientific lens, the concepts of this widely consumed drug are examined to show its merits and refute misconceptions. The analyses also explored the known and projected effects of cannabis on normal body processes and what happens when those processes break down. There was a real effort to make sure there was no impression of discouraging or encouraging people to take cannabis. Instead, this book is meant to empower the general public with fundamental scientific knowledge and understanding. This knowledge will help them make better decisions before experimenting with this drug.

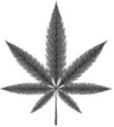

16

Parents, teachers, healthcare providers, community leaders, and educators can use the information in this book to educate their communities about the dangers and benefits of cannabis. By educating their communities about cannabis, these people are helping to create a more informed decision-making process and a better understanding of the drug's effects. In the book, parents will discover the risks associated with cannabis use and discuss them with their kids. Parents can also help their kids make wise decisions if they decide to consume it. In 2019, about 48.2 million people, or 18% of Americans, were reported to have used cannabis at least once. That's a lot of people, so if your kid says they're heading to a 'study group,' double-check.

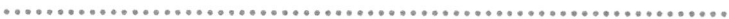

It's imperative to understand the effects of cannabis on your body, as it can have both positive and negative impacts on your overall health. For instance, research has shown that cannabis can help with pain relief, reduce inflammation, and even the symptoms of certain mental health conditions like PTSD and depression. However, there're also potential risks associated with cannabis use, such as increased risk of anxiety and paranoia, impaired coordination, and decreased academic performance.

Therefore, it's essential to be aware of both the potential benefits and risks of cannabis use before deciding to incorporate it into your lifestyle. For instance, research suggests that there may be a link between cannabis use and the development of psychosis in some individuals, so it's recommended that those with any pre-existing mental health conditions consult a doctor before using cannabis. Additionally, people should be mindful of the possible legal ramifications of using cannabis, as it's still a controlled substance in many countries and territories.

17

Other proven therapeutic benefits of cannabis include reduction in nausea and vomiting, and improving muscle stiffness and spasms in people with multiple sclerosis. This's not to say that cannabis is a cure for these health problems, but when there's no alternative, cannabis has been shown to help. It may not provide a cure, but it can improve the quality of life when traditional therapeutics fail.

While cannabis has been shown to help with several medical issues, it has drawbacks. Cannabis can negatively affect short-term memory, judgment, and motor skills. It can also lead to anxiety and paranoia, especially in high doses. Some long-term effects of cannabis use include risks to lung health, mental health problems, and lower life satisfaction. As comedian Louis C.K. once said, "Drugs are so good that they'll ruin your life."

If you find more information critical about cannabis pre-

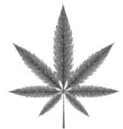

sented throughout this book than information promoting cannabis, that's not by design. We don't have enough research on the risks and benefits; however, we can infer both from what we know about the extensive research on other drugs as a guide. If something is wrong with your car, you can open it up, figure out what's wrong, and fix the problem. You can also try one solution; if it doesn't work, you move on to the next possible solution.

Human beings, on the other hand, require a high degree of certainty when it comes to diagnosing and treating medical conditions. It'd be best if you were certain because some mistakes can cost a patient their life and a doctor their license. Doctors use past studies, history, and outcomes of similar treatments to avoid malpractice lawsuits and predict how their treatment will affect each patient.

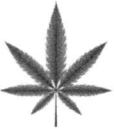

18

Since you can't test each medicine on every patient, past studies, other drugs, and possible side effects are all used to extrapolate the impact of the medication on each patient. The same holds for cannabis. It may be decades before we understand cannabis entirely in all its forms. For now, we have only user stories, small studies, and dozens of books about other drugs. At this point, we can only use this information to extrapolate the scientific effects and complications of cannabis use in any form.

While the drugs may not be the same, they share some interesting similarities in their chemistry and pharmacology that make the comparison easier. It's critical to note that while cannabis has been used for centuries, current research on its effects is still limited. This makes it difficult to draw definitive conclusions about its potential benefits or risks.

We can't discuss everything in every detail on the topic of cannabis. Instead, we'll focus on some significant points and what can be simplified for those with little to no medical background. Please remember that the

book was written for people without a solid scientific foundation. Hence, some topics and concepts needed to be more concise. We'll start with what's known on the surface about cannabis smoking. We'll then move on to more complicated topics such as metabolism, law, economics, social impact, and some associated problems. We'll also discuss the different forms of cannabis consumption, such as smoking, vaping, and edibles, and how they may affect your body differently. It's essential to understand the various ways cannabis can be consumed and the potential effects and complications they may have.

There're references at the end for further reading and a glossary of terms for brief meanings of the main scientific terms used throughout this book.

A journey of a thousand miles begins with one step, so let's take that first step now.

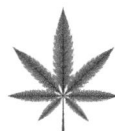

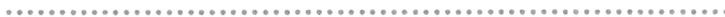

In the words of the late Dr. Milton H. Erickson, a renowned psychiatrist and author, much of what we do in life is influenced by unconscious decisions. Take a moment to reflect on meaningful moments, like your first kiss, selecting a best friend, falling in love, or deciding on a life path. These decisions may have seemed inconsequential at the time. Still, they have profoundly impacted your life, often in ways you may not have fully recognized.

Recall, if you can, the exact moment you chose your favourite colour or when thoughts of sex first entered your mind. The specifics of those moments likely elude your memory. These decisions are often unconsciously guided by our instincts and natural inclinations. They become part of an unconscious thought process that develops its own internal logic until, one day, and we become conscious of those choices. This awareness may come days, weeks, months, years, or even decades later.

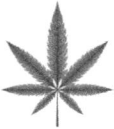

Whether the decisions are significant or seemingly trivial, the cognitive process behind them operates similarly: unconscious ideas and reasoning that lead to conscious choices. We may believe that we make these decisions through careful deliberation and planning. Still, our unconscious impulses and instincts play a substantial role.

20

This is how the human mind naturally operates. However, find yourself spending excessive time grappling with decisions like choosing a favourite colour or obsessing over matters of sex. It may be beneficial to seek professional assistance. While this book does not offer a straightforward solution to such dilemmas, it can provide insights into human nature and how the brain functions.

Understanding the unconscious processes that influence our decision-making can shed light on our behaviours and motivations. By gaining this knowledge, you can better understand yourself and the mechanisms at work within your mind. Remember, this book serves as a tool to enhance understanding, but seeking professional help when needed is always a valuable option.

It all starts with a puff

Cannabis is a plant that has been used for various purposes for thousands of years. Known by many names such as marijuana, weed, pot, grass, herb, ganja, reefer, dope, Mary Jane, hash, hashish, hemp, sinsemilla, skunk, or bud, this plant has been utilized for both medicinal and recreational purposes, as well as for its fibres and oils.

Cannabis has been used to create paper, rope, and textiles, and its psychoactive properties have been enjoyed by many. **Psychoactive properties** mean cannabis can alter how your brain work, leading to changes in your thoughts, feelings, and perceptions. This's why some people find using cannabis enjoyable or relaxing. It has also been used for spiritual and religious ceremonies.

Some scientific studies have suggested that cannabis may have potential health benefits. For example, it has been found to relieve pain, reduce **inflammation**, and even alleviate symptoms of **anxiety** and **depression**. These potential benefits have led to increased interest in researching cannabis and its compounds for medicinal purposes.

However, it is essential to note that cannabis isn't without its risks. The effects of cannabis on your brain can be both positive and negative. On the negative side, cannabis has been shown to impair memory and learning abilities, slow reaction times, and induce **paranoia** and anxiety in some individuals. These effects can vary depending on factors such as the dose consumed, method of consumption, and your unique biology.

In addition, regular and heavy use of cannabis is associated with an increased risk of developing **psychotic disorders**, such as **schizophrenia**. According to a

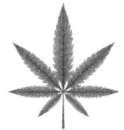

21

recent study that included 36 different studies, 49% of cannabis users will experience **psychosis** at some point in their lifetime. So if you're considering trying cannabis, remember you might have a 50/50 chance of going crazy!

While these findings are significant, it's important to remember that not everyone who uses cannabis will develop these disorders. However, it's essential to be aware of the potential risks and to make informed decisions regarding cannabis use. It's worth noting that the statistics mentioned earlier regarding the risk of psychosis are based on research findings and may vary depending on the population studied and other factors.

In recent decades, cannabis use has become increasingly controversial, with opinions divided on its potential benefits and risks. While the possible effects of cannabis use remain a source of debate, one thing is for sure - it has the potential to change your life for better or worse dramatically!

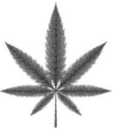

22

Proponents of cannabis use point to studies that suggest it may have medical benefits, such as reducing inflammation and pain, improving sleep, and helping with anxiety and depression. However, opponents point to evidence suggesting cannabis use can lead to **addiction**, memory problems, and other mental health issues like psychosis.

Despite its widespread use, much is still unclear about this plant's effects on the human body. While there may be health risks associated with cannabis use, it's pertinent to recognize that a considerable amount of research still needs to be done to understand its full range of effects. For instance, further research is required to understand how cannabis affects different age groups and interacts with other substances, such as alcohol and nicotine. As Charles Darwin once wrote: "Ignorance more frequently begets confidence than does knowledge: it is those who know little, not those who know much, who so positively assert that this or that problem will never be solved by science."

Studies have shown that certain compounds found in cannabis, such as **THC** (delta-9-tetrahydrocannabinol) and **CBD** (cannabidiol), may have **anti-inflammatory** and **analgesic properties**, which could potentially help with conditions like inflammation and **chronic pain**, respectively. Additionally, some individuals have reported improved sleep quality and reduced anxiety and depression symptoms after using cannabis. However, it's important to note that the effects can vary from person to person, and more research is needed to establish the optimal dosages, formulations, and long-term effects.

Regular and heavy cannabis use has been linked to an increased risk of developing **dependence** or addiction, particularly in individuals who start using it at a young age. Furthermore, cannabis use can impair **cognitive function**, especially in areas related to memory, attention, and decision-making. It's worth mentioning that these effects are more pronounced with high levels of THC, the **psychoactive compound** in cannabis.

23

The legal status of cannabis has significantly impacted the knowledge and understanding of the plant. The long-standing illegal status of cannabis has created various barriers that hindered **scientific research** and limited access to reliable information. These restrictions have had implications on multiple fronts, including funding, approval processes, and availability of resources for researchers.

The stigma surrounding cannabis has been perpetuated by its illegal status in most parts of the world, making it challenging for researchers to obtain funding. Many funding sources, including government agencies and research institutions, have been hes-

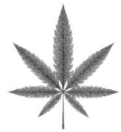

itant to support cannabis-related research due to the legal and social complexities associated with the plant. This lack of funding has restricted the number and scale of studies, limiting our understanding of cannabis and its effects.

Additionally, the legal classification of cannabis as a Schedule 1 drug in some countries, including the United States, has imposed strict regulations on its research. Schedule 1 substances have a high potential for abuse and no recognized medical value. This classification has created significant obstacles for researchers in obtaining the necessary permissions and licenses to study cannabis and its potential benefits or risks. The stringent regulations have made it difficult to conduct large-scale clinical trials or access standardized research-grade cannabis, further impeding scientific progress.

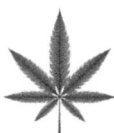

24

The limited availability of research opportunities has resulted in a scarcity of objective data and scientific evidence on cannabis. Instead, **anecdotal evidence** and individual experiences have often filled the void, leading to a fragmented understanding of its effects. While personal accounts provide valuable insights, they may only sometimes reflect the full range of potential outcomes or apply only to a few.

However, it's important to note that the landscape is evolving. As attitudes and laws surrounding cannabis change, there's a growing interest in conducting rigorous scientific research to fill the knowledge gaps. Efforts are being made to expand access to research funding, ease regulatory restrictions, and promote **evidence-based** approaches to understanding cannabis.

By fostering an environment that encourages scientific exploration and open dialogue, we can move away from the symbolic "dark ages" and work towards a

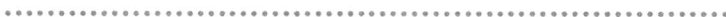

more comprehensive understanding of cannabis and its effects on the human body.

Through rigorous scientific investigation, we can gather reliable evidence and make informed decisions. As with any **scientific inquiry**, it's crucial to remain open to new findings and be willing to adjust your understanding based on your accumulation of knowledge. **Scientific discovery** often involves asking questions, formulating hypotheses, conducting experiments, and analyzing data to draw meaningful conclusions. This iterative process allows us to refine our understanding and uncover new insights.

In the case of cannabis, ongoing research aims to address various unanswered questions. This includes investigating its potential therapeutic applications, exploring its impact on different populations, and understanding the possible interactions with other substances. It's worth noting that the scientific method is designed to challenge existing assumptions and continuously refine our understanding. It encourages a humble approach to knowledge, recognizing there's always more to discover. As we strive to uncover the truth about cannabis, it's vital to approach the topic with an open mind and rely on **scientific evidence** to guide our understanding.

25

When considering cannabis as a treatment option, balancing the potential benefits and risks is crucial. While some individuals have reported finding relief from various ailments, it's essential to approach cannabis use with caution. The increased speculation about adverse effects such as addiction, impaired cognitive function, and a higher risk of mental health disorders shouldn't be ignored.

Consulting a medical professional before embarking on any cannabis-based treatment plan is highly recommended. **Medical professionals** can provide personalized advice based on your specific health cir-

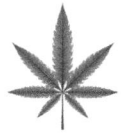

cumstances and help weigh the potential risks and benefits. It's like crossing a busy intersection – even if the destination seems promising, taking the time to look both ways ensures your safety.

Considering the long-term effects of cannabis use is particularly important. Some individuals may experience short-term relief, but the risks associated with prolonged use may outweigh the initial benefits. You can make informed decisions that prioritize your overall well-being by seeking **medical advice**. Benjamin Franklin's timeless quote, "An ounce of prevention is worth a pound of cure," aptly reminds us of the significance of preventive measures. By being proactive and cautious, you can prevent future complications and make choices that align with your overall health goals.

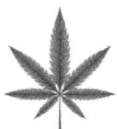

Understanding the potential benefits and risks of cannabis is essential for all individuals involved in its use, including patients, doctors, suppliers, and regulators. **Healthcare providers** who recommend cannabis as a treatment option should comprehensively understand its **pharmacology**, potential interactions with other medications, and the specific **medical conditions** for which it may be suitable. They play a critical role in assessing the patient's individual circumstances and determining the appropriateness of cannabis as part of their treatment plan.

26

Suppliers and **manufacturers** of cannabis-based products also bear the responsibility of ensuring quality, safety, and accurate labelling. This includes providing transparent information about the potency and composition of their products and adhering to appropriate manufacturing and quality control standards.

When it comes to recreational cannabis use, there're essential considerations to keep in mind. Unlike **medicinal cannabis**, which focuses on maximizing **therapeutic** benefits, **recreational** use carries different risks. The responsibility for educating consumers about the potential dangers of cannabis consumption often falls on the suppliers. However, it's vital to recognize that suppliers may have a conflict of interest, as they're driven by profit and may downplay the risks associated with cannabis.

In this context, **government regulations** are crucial in safeguarding consumers from potential harm. These regulations establish guidelines for **product safety**, labelling, and **responsible marketing practices**. While the extent to which governments act in the best interests of the people may vary, regulations are necessary to protect consumers from unscrupulous suppliers and ensure transparency in the cannabis market.

Nevertheless, it's ultimately up to individuals to take responsibility for their well-being and make informed decisions. Educating yourself about the risks associated with cannabis use is crucial. This includes being aware of potential short-term and long-term health risks, such as **respiratory issues** from smoking cannabis or the potential for addiction. It also involves understanding the legal implications, as cannabis laws vary across jurisdictions, and possession or use may lead to legal consequences.

27

Approaching recreational cannabis use without adequate knowledge or research is akin to navigating a minefield. It's essential to proceed cautiously, know your boundaries, and be well-informed about the potential dangers. Taking the time to educate yourself about the risks associated with cannabis can help you make responsible choices and minimize the likelihood of experiencing adverse consequences.

With the legalization of cannabis in certain regions, there's now a more significant opportunity for researchers to delve deeper into the study of this plant and its impact on the human body. This shift in the regulatory landscape opens doors for more comprehensive investigations that can contribute to our understanding of cannabis.

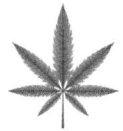

The current research efforts aim to address important questions regarding cannabis use and its effects on various aspects of human health. One prominent area of study is the relationship between cannabis and mental health. Researchers are examining the potential links between cannabis use and conditions such as anxiety, depression, and psychosis. These studies involve analyzing large datasets, conducting **longitudinal studies**, and exploring the underlying mechanisms to better understand the potential risks and benefits associated with cannabis use.

Furthermore, researchers are investigating the therapeutic potential of cannabis for managing chronic pain and other medical conditions. Studies are exploring the effectiveness of **cannabinoids** in alleviating symptoms and improving quality of life. This research includes **clinical trials**, **observational studies**, and laboratory experiments to provide a more comprehensive understanding of the potential medical applications of cannabis.

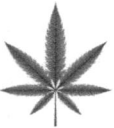

28

By accumulating scientific evidence through rigorous research, policymakers and regulatory bodies can make more informed decisions regarding the use, distribution, and accessibility of cannabis. This evidence-based approach can guide the development of public health policies that strike a balance between maximizing potential benefits and minimizing potential risks.

It's important to note that ongoing research is still necessary to uncover the full range of positive and negative effects associated with cannabis use. As our understanding of cannabis continues to evolve, it's vital to approach the subject with curiosity and willingness to explore new information. As more studies are conducted and scientific knowledge accumulates, a more transparent and comprehensive picture of cannabis and its potential risks and benefits will emerge. This continuous process of dis-

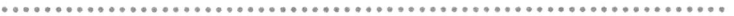

covery and understanding is like an **archaeological excavation**, where each layer of evidence reveals new insights and contributes to our overall knowledge. This includes understanding the individual factors that may influence how cannabis affects each person differently.

It's valuable to recognize that scientific research takes time and requires a rigorous process to ensure accurate and reliable findings. As more studies are conducted, and evidence accumulates, our understanding of cannabis will continue to improve.

It's also worth noting that open and honest discussions surrounding cannabis can help promote a balanced perspective. Engaging in conversations with healthcare professionals, researchers, and others with expertise in the field can provide valuable insights and ensure that decisions regarding cannabis use are based on reliable information.

Remember, staying informed and open to new information allows a more comprehensive understanding of cannabis and its potential impact on individuals and society.

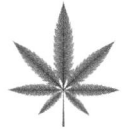

Have you ever stopped to think about the reasons behind your quirky behaviour? Do you jump into things headfirst and figure out the logic later, or do you carefully plan your every move like a chess master? And what happens when you realize you've goofed? Do you stubbornly stick to your blunder, or do you admit defeat and course-correct like a seasoned captain?

Let's face it; we're not all-knowing superheroes. We all mess up, and we all have our blind spots. None of us have a monopoly on wisdom, which is why it's wise to lend an ear to the advice of others. Taking a moment to pause and reflect before you leap can save you from tripping over your own ego. You may think you're the most brilliant cookie in the jar, but there's always something to learn from your fellow cookie monsters.

It's crucial to keep an open mind and consider different perspectives. Even if you're not sold on someone's suggestions, giving them a fair shake and pondering their words of wisdom doesn't hurt. These questions might be pesky little critters, but they may hold some profound truth.

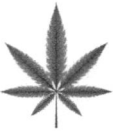

30

Awareness of your mental machinery and questioning your actions can be eye-opening. By practicing mindfulness and reflection, you can make better choices and avoid epic faceplants. So, next time you're about to unleash your grand plan, take a moment to ponder. Think deeply, explore alternatives, and remember that hasty decisions can leave you swimming in regret.

Firing Up The Bags Of Wind

The Three Standard Methods Of Cannabis Consumption

Cannabis consumption comes in various forms, but the most common method is smoking. It's like the classic choice of how to enjoy your favourite treat. Just like some people prefer to eat their ice cream right out of the cone, many cannabis enthusiasts enjoy the convenience and immediate effects of smoking. All you need are the proper rolling papers, a little skill in rolling it up and a lighter, and you puff that magic dragon. It's like a DIY project on the go, crafting your own little smokeable creation.

But hold on; there's more to the story! As technology advances and our understanding of cannabis grows, alternative methods of consumption have emerged. **Vaporizers** and **edibles** are gaining popularity among cannabis users. Think of them as high-tech options for the more discerning enthusiasts.

31

Vaporizers, or "vapes" for short, have become trendy in some parts of the world. They heat the cannabis to a temperature that releases the active compounds without producing as much smoke. It's like using a sophisticated gadget to extract the plant's essence. However, it's important to note that long-term and excessive use of vaporizers may have some side effects, so moderation is key. It's like having a fancy new toy, but you must be mindful of how much you play with it to avoid unintended consequences.

Now let's talk about edibles, the culinary adventure of cannabis consumption. Instead of rolling up a joint or puffing on a vape, some people choose to incorporate cannabis into their food. Brownies, cookies, gummies, you name it! It's like taking your favourite ingredients and adding a "special twist." But here's the catch:

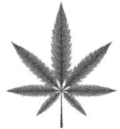

making edibles requires time and effort. Unless you find pre-made edibles, you'll need to dedicate some kitchen time to infuse cannabis into your favourite recipes. And let's be honest, not everyone is up for that cooking or baking challenge, especially when looking for a quick high.

While vaporizers and edibles offer different experiences and potential advantages, smoking remains the go-to method for many cannabis users. It's like sticking to the tried-and-true classics. But hey, it's always good to keep an open mind and explore different options. Who knows, you might discover a new favourite way to enjoy cannabis.

From Your Breath To Your Circulatory System

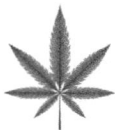

When you smoke cannabis, the smoke enters your lungs and makes its way to a crucial part of your lungs called the **alveolus**. You can think of your lungs as an upside-down tree, where the trunk is your **trachea** (throat), and the branches are the **bronchi**. The alveoli, on the other hand, are like the leaves of a tree. Just as water travels up the trunk and branches to reach the leaves, when you inhale, oxygen or cannabis smoke follows a similar path from your throat to your alveolus.

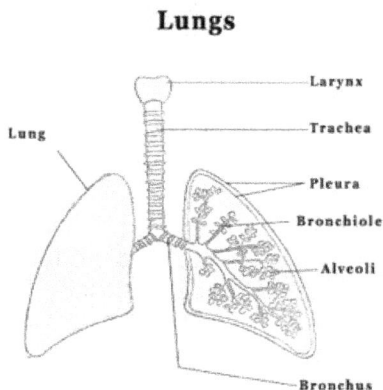

32

Lungs

- Larynx
- Lung
- Trachea
- Pleura
- Bronchiole
- Alveoli
- Bronchus

The alveoli, or leaves of the respiratory tree, are tiny air sacs where gas exchange occurs. When you breathe in oxygen, it diffuses across the walls of the alveoli and into your bloodstream. This's how oxygen reaches all parts of your body to support vital functions. In the case of cannabis smoke, the active compounds in the smoke also enter the bloodstream through the alveoli.

It's important to note that smoking cannabis involves inhaling smoke, which contains various chemicals and particles. While the alveoli are efficient at absorbing gases, the smoke from cannabis may negatively affect your **respiratory system**. Research has linked smoking cannabis to respiratory issues, such as coughing, **bronchitis**, and lung damage. That's why alternative methods of consumption, like vaporizers or edibles, are gaining popularity as they offer potential advantages in reducing the potential harm associated with smoking.

When oxygen gets into your blood, it binds to red blood cells that will then transport this oxygen to your tissues. When oxygen reaches your tissues, it can then be used to burn the food you eat to produce energy, just like a car burns gasoline or diesel to work. You'll then use this energy for anything, from sprinting to the most intrinsic metabolic properties like **digestion** and synthesizing **hormones** and other biochemicals. However, cannabis is unlike oxygen; your body doesn't require it for **metabolic processes**. Thus, cannabis has a very different path of use by your body after it's absorbed into your blood.

What is cannabis?

Cannabis is a **herb**, which means a natural plant containing up to dozens of active **biochemical ingredients**. We don't know most of these other chemicals and what they do to someone who smokes cannabis. However, we have isolated and studied the com-

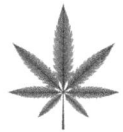

33

pound tetrahydrocannabinol, also known as THC. THC interacts with specific receptors in your brain called **cannabinoid receptors**. These receptors are part of a complex system known as the **endocannabinoid system**, which regulates various **physiological functions**.

When THC binds to cannabinoid receptors, it can affect the release of certain **neurotransmitters**, which are chemical messengers in your brain. This interaction of THC and cannabinoid receptors can lead to various effects on mood, **cognition, perception**, and **sensation**, which is why people use cannabis for recreational purposes.

It's important to remember that the effects of cannabis can vary depending on factors such as the **strain of cannabis**, the method of consumption, the **dose**, and an individual's unique **physiology**. Some people may experience relaxation and euphoria, while others may feel **anxious** or **paranoid**. These effects can also be influenced by the presence of other compounds in cannabis, such as CBD (cannabidiol), which has different properties.

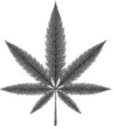

34

When cannabis is smoked or vaporized, the heat causes THC to be released in the form of vapour or smoke. This vapour or smoke contains THC molecules, which are then inhaled into your lungs. The large surface area of your lungs allows for rapid absorption of THC into your bloodstream, facilitating its quick distribution throughout your body.

Because of this quick absorption, the effects of cannabis can be felt within minutes of inhalation. This immediate onset is one of the reasons why smoking or vaporizing cannabis is popular among **recreational users**.

What happens when cannabis enters your brain?

One of the outcomes of THC binding to CB1 receptors is the release of neurotransmitters, including dopamine. **Dopamine** is a neurotransmitter that is associated with your brain's reward system. It plays a crucial role in regulating pleasure, motivation, and reinforcement. When THC activates dopamine release, it can contribute to the feelings of euphoria and reward commonly experienced when using cannabis.

In addition to dopamine, THC's interaction with **CB1 receptors** can also affect other neurotransmitter systems, such as **serotonin** and **norepinephrine**, which can influence mood, cognition, and other physiological processes. These interactions are part of the complex mechanism by which THC exerts its psychoactive effects.

It's important to note that while THC's interaction with CB1 receptors can produce pleasurable effects, it can also have other effects on cognition, memory, **coordination**, and overall brain function depending on dose, individual sensitivity, and previous cannabis use. The presence of CB1 receptors in your **hippocampus** plays a significant role in the effects of THC on memory and cognition. The hippocampus is responsible for the formation and retrieval of memories, as well as the regulation of emotions.

When THC binds to CB1 receptors in your hippocampus, it can disrupt the normal functioning of this region. This interference can temporarily impair memory formation, recall, and attention. It can also affect the ability to learn and retain new information. These effects may manifest as difficulty remembering recent events or maintaining focus on tasks requiring cognitive effort. Additionally, THC's activation of CB1 receptors in your hippocampus can modulate emotional responses. This can result in relaxation, euphoria, and altered mood. However, it's important to note that the

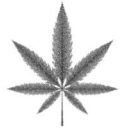

impact of THC on emotions can vary among individuals, and some individuals may experience heightened anxiety or negative emotions in certain situations.

What causes the variations in cannabis effects in different people?

The effects of cannabis can vary significantly among individuals due to many factors. These factors can include individual differences in **metabolism, genetic makeup, tolerance**, and overall health. Factors such as **strain potency**, method of consumption, and dosage can also contribute to the variability in effects.

The strain of cannabis refers to the specific variety or genetic makeup of the plant, which can have different levels of cannabinoids, including THC and CBD, as well as other compounds. Different strains can produce varying effects, with some strains being associated with more relaxing or **sedating effects**. In contrast, others may be more energizing or uplifting.

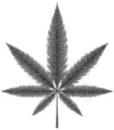

36

The method of consumption also plays a role in the onset and duration of effects. Smoking or vaporizing cannabis typically results in a faster onset of effects, as the cannabinoids are rapidly absorbed into your bloodstream through your lungs. On the other hand, when cannabis is consumed orally, such as through edibles, the effects may take longer to manifest but can also last longer.

Moreover, individual factors such as body size and composition can influence how cannabis is metabolized and distributed in your body. Concurrent drug use, including prescribed medications or other substances, can also interact with cannabis and potentially impact its effects. Furthermore, an individual's personal history with cannabis use, including frequency, duration, and any previous experiences, can influence how they respond to the drug.

It's important to note that excessive or prolonged use of cannabis, especially at high doses, can increase the risk of adverse effects. These may include increased anxiety, paranoia, impaired memory and cognitive functions, and potential dependence or addiction. Understanding these potential risks and using cannabis responsibly and in moderation is crucial.

What is respiration?

Respiration is how living organisms, including humans, obtain energy from the environment. It's a vital process that allows your body to convert fuel into usable energy to support various functions and activities.

In mammals, including humans, respiration involves two main stages: external respiration and internal respiration. Let's take a closer look at each of these stages:

1. **External Respiration**:
    External respiration occurs in your lungs. It is the process of exchanging gases between the external environment and your body.
    During external respiration, you inhale oxygen-rich air and exhale carbon dioxide, which is a waste product of **cellular metabolism**.
    When you inhale, air enters your respiratory system through your nose or mouth. It then travels down your trachea, which branches into smaller tubes called bronchi. The bronchi further divide into even smaller tubes called **bronchioles**, which eventually lead to tiny air sacs called alveoli. The alveoli are the site of gas exchange. They're surrounded by blood vessels, and it's in the alveoli that oxygen from the inhaled air diffuses into your bloodstream. In contrast, carbon dioxide, a waste product produced by

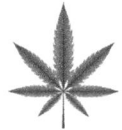

37

your cells, diffuses out of your bloodstream into the alveoli. This exchange of gases occurs due to differences in their concentration across the thin walls of the alveoli and blood vessels.

2. **Internal Respiration**: Internal respiration takes place in the cells of your body. It involves the exchange of gases between your blood and your cells, where oxygen is utilized by your cells to produce energy and carbon dioxide. Carbon dioxide is a by-product of cellular metabolism.

Oxygen's Journey After Leaving Your Lungs

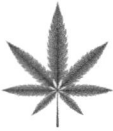

38

After oxygen from the inhaled air enters your bloodstream in your lungs, it binds to **hemoglobin**, a protein in red blood cells that carries oxygen throughout your body. Once attached to oxygen, this blood is now called oxygenated blood. **Oxygenated blood** is then transported to various tissues and organs throughout your body.

Capillaries are the smallest blood vessels where gas exchange occurs between your blood and cells. In your capillaries, oxygen diffuses out of your bloodstream and enters your cells, participating in a series of chemical reactions called cellular respiration. These reactions break down fuel molecules, such as glucose, to produce **adenosine triphosphate** (ATP), the energy currency of cells.

During cellular respiration, oxygen reacts with glucose to release energy, carbon dioxide, and water. The energy released is used to perform various cellular functions, such as muscle contraction, **nerve signalling**, and maintenance of body temperature. The waste product carbon dioxide is transported back to your

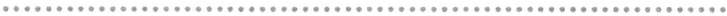

lungs through the bloodstream and is exhaled during external respiration.

What Is Dalton's Law Of Partial Pressure?

Normal gaseous exchange in respiration is a crucial process by which your body obtains oxygen from the environment and eliminates carbon dioxide. This process occurs in your lungs and is driven by differences in the **partial pressures** of these gases, as explained by Dalton's law of partial pressures.

Dalton's law states that the total pressure exerted by a mixture of gases is equal to the sum of the pressures exerted by each individual gas, known as its partial pressure. In respiration, the partial pressures of oxygen and carbon dioxide play a significant role.

When you inhale, fresh air enters your respiratory system and reaches the alveoli in your lungs. The oxygen concentration in your alveoli is higher than that in your blood, creating a partial pressure gradient. This difference in partial pressures causes oxygen to diffuse from your alveoli into your bloodstream, down the pressure gradient.

39

Oxygen molecules then bind to hemoglobin in red blood cells, allowing efficient transportation of oxygen to tissues and organs throughout your body. At the same time, carbon dioxide, produced as a waste product of cellular metabolism, diffuses from your bloodstream into your alveoli, where its partial pressure is lower. Again, a pressure gradient allows this movement of carbon dioxide, which allows for its elimination when you exhale.

The exchange of oxygen and carbon dioxide between your alveoli and your bloodstream is facilitated by thin walls, a large surface area in your alveoli, and the network of capillaries surrounding them. These structural features promote the efficient diffusion of gases across your respiratory membrane.

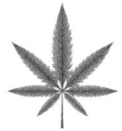

By maintaining an appropriate balance of oxygen and carbon dioxide in your bloodstream, gaseous exchange in respiration ensures that your cells receive the oxygen they need for energy production and that waste carbon dioxide is efficiently removed from your body.

What Happens When Partial Pressures Are Disturbed?

According to Dalton's law of partial pressures, these gases are all kept at constant pressure so that your lungs neither collapse nor expand out of proportion. The pressure of each of the gases is a "part" of the total pressure in your lungs, hence the partial pressure of that particular gas. At equilibrium, the combined sum of the partial pressures in your lungs equals the **standard atmospheric pressure**, 760 mmHg.

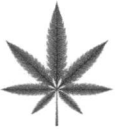

Since these gases are kept at constant pressure, if the pressure of one of the gases goes up, the pressure of the other gas should come down, and vice versa. This means that if the partial pressure of oxygen is 600mmHg, then the partial pressure of carbon dioxide has to be 160mmHg. If the partial pressure of oxygen in your lungs drops to 200mmHg, the partial pressure of carbon dioxide will have to increase to 560mmHg. The total partial pressure in your lungs must stay constant. Another way to look at this is if the normal pressure of all gases in normal lungs is 760mmHg, and 50% of that is from oxygen while the other half is from carbon dioxide, the addition of another gas like carbon monoxide will lower the amount of normal gases in your lungs in order to maintain the constant pressure in your lungs.

Thus, the addition of carbon monoxide will lower the pressures of both carbon dioxide and oxygen. Mathematically, suppose you add 20% of the total pressure in your lungs with carbon monoxide. In that case, the partial pressures of oxygen and car-

40

bon dioxide may decrease from 50% to 40% each to add up to 100%.

Remember, oxygen is taken in during inhalation, and its partial pressure in your alveoli increases, creating a pressure gradient that allows oxygen to diffuse into your bloodstream. Simultaneously, carbon dioxide, which has a higher partial pressure in your bloodstream, diffuses from your blood into your alveoli to be exhaled during exhalation.

This continuous exchange of gases between your alveoli and your blood ensures that oxygen is supplied to your tissues and carbon dioxide is removed from your body. The process relies on the principles of **diffusion** and the differences in partial pressures to achieve efficient gas exchange.
In summary, during cellular respiration, oxygen combines with glucose (a sugar molecule obtained from the breakdown of carbohydrates) within your cells to produce energy in the form of adenosine triphosphate (ATP), the primary energy currency of cells. This process occurs in the **mitochondria**, often called the "powerhouses" of your cells.

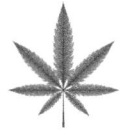

41

The reaction of oxygen with glucose in cellular respiration produces carbon dioxide and water as by-products. Carbon dioxide enters your bloodstream as a waste product and is transported back to your lungs through the venous system.

Once in your lungs, carbon dioxide is exchanged for oxygen through pulmonary gas exchange. Carbon dioxide diffuses from your blood into your alveoli, while oxygen diffuses from your alveoli into your blood. Carbon dioxide is then expelled from your lungs during exhalation, completing the cycle of gaseous exchange.

This process of cellular respiration and pulmonary gas exchange ensures a continuous supply of oxygen to your cells for energy production and carbon dioxide removal, maintaining a balance in your body's respiratory function.

How Do Your Alveoli Participate In Respiration?

The alveoli, tiny air sacs located at the ends of the bronchioles in your lungs, play a crucial role in the gaseous exchange process. Their thin walls comprise a single layer of flattened cells known as **squamous epithelial** cells. This thinness allows gases like oxygen and carbon dioxide to diffuse easily across the **alveolar membrane**.

The large surface area of your alveoli is made possible by their numerous small spherical shapes and the presence of millions of alveoli in your lungs. This extensive surface area provides a vast area for gas exchange between the alveoli and the surrounding capillaries.

How Do Your Capillaries Participate In Respiration?

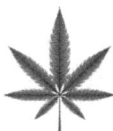

42

Capillaries are tiny blood vessels with thin walls that form a dense network surrounding your alveoli. The walls of your capillaries are also thin, consisting of a single layer of **endothelial cells**. This thinness facilitates the proximity of your capillaries to your alveoli, allowing for efficient diffusion of gases between your blood and your alveoli.

During inhalation, oxygen-rich air enters your alveoli, and the oxygen concentration in your alveoli becomes higher than in the surrounding capillaries. As a result, oxygen diffuses from your alveoli into your capillaries, binding to hemoglobin in red blood cells for transport to your body tissues.

On the other hand, carbon dioxide, a waste product produced by your metabolism, has a higher concentration in your capillaries than in your alveoli. This concentration gradient causes carbon dioxide to diffuse from your capillaries into your alveoli, where it is expelled during exhalation.

How Does Cannabis Affect Normal Gas Exchange?

When you smoke cannabis or any other substance, **combustion** occurs, producing smoke that contains a mixture of gases, **particulate matter**, and chemicals. This smoke can irritate your respiratory system, causing symptoms such as coughing, **wheezing**, and **shortness of breath**. Prolonged exposure to smoke, whether from cannabis or other sources, can potentially lead to **chronic respiratory problems**.

Furthermore, the combustion of cannabis releases harmful by-products, such as carbon monoxide and **tar**, which can have detrimental effects on your lungs. Carbon monoxide reduces the ability of blood to carry oxygen, potentially leading to oxygen deprivation in your tissues. Tar, a sticky substance, can accumulate in your airways and lungs, contributing to respiratory issues and increasing the risk of **chronic bronchitis** and other lung diseases.

It's also worth mentioning that long-term cannabis smoking has been associated with an increased risk of respiratory infections and the development of lung cancer, similar to the risks associated with tobacco smoking. However, it's important to note that the risks may vary.
Oxygen is essential for your energy production and overall functioning. When the amount of oxygen available to your body decreases, it can have significant implications for health and well-being.

43

What Is Hypoxia?

When there's a decrease in the amount of oxygen available to your body, it can result in a condition called hypoxia. **Hypoxia** occurs when there is insufficient oxygen supply to meet your body's metabolic demands. This can happen for various reasons, including reduced environmental oxygen, impaired lung function, or inadequate circulation of oxygenated blood.

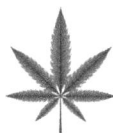

The symptoms of hypoxia can vary depending on the severity and duration of oxygen deprivation. Mild hypoxia may cause fatigue, headaches, dizziness, and shortness of breath. As the oxygen supply continues to decrease, more severe symptoms can develop, including confusion, rapid heartbeat, chest pain, and **cyanosis** (bluish discoloration of the skin and mucous membranes).

In prolonged or severe oxygen deprivation, such as chronic respiratory diseases or cardiovascular conditions, your organs, including your heart, can be adversely affected. Inadequate oxygen supply to your heart muscle can lead to **heart failure**. In this condition, the heart's ability to pump blood efficiently is severely compromised.

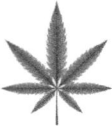

Decreasing the amount of oxygen in your body is like running a car with less fuel. Eventually, the engine will grind to a halt, and your vehicle will no longer be able to move. The same can be said for your body – a decrease in the amount of oxygen available will have dire consequences for your health and well-being.

44

Did you know that deep-diving mammals have several adaptations that allow them to stay underwater for long periods without breathing? These adaptations include filling their lungs and exchanging 90% of their air in each breath, high blood volume, and blood chemistry, allowing for more excellent oxygen retention. While humans don't possess these specific adaptations, our bodies have their own remarkable mechanisms for maintaining adequate oxygen levels during normal respiration.

What Is Homocysteine?

Another potential consequence of hypoxia is increased levels of a substance called homocysteine in your blood. **Homocysteine** is an **amino acid** that, when present in high levels, is associated with an increased risk of various health issues, including **blood clots**. Blood clots can be particularly concerning when they travel to critical organs like your brain, leading to strokes, or when they affect the heart's blood vessels, leading to **heart attacks**.

It's well-established that smoking, including inhaling toxic gases from any source, increases the risk of various health issues, including heart attacks and strokes. The tobacco industry has indeed taught us valuable lessons about the detrimental effects of smoking on **cardiovascular health**. Smoking tobacco has been linked to the development of **atherosclerosis** (narrowing and hardening of the arteries), which can lead to heart attacks or strokes.

What's The Relationship Between Smoking And Ocps?

When it comes to combining smoking with certain medications, such as **Oral Contraceptive Pills** (OCPs), it's crucial to consider the potential interactions and risks involved. OCPs themselves have been associated with a slight increase in the risk of blood clots. When smoking is combined with OCP use, the risk of blood clots, including those leading to heart attacks or strokes, may be elevated. To this day, women are routinely advised to stay away from smoking while taking OCPs. Some women prefer to keep smoking and avoid OCPs, but that's their decision; freedom of choice. Either way, smoking and taking OCPs should never be done together, even within several weeks of each other.

Estrogen promotes the production of certain blood **clotting factors**, which can lead to an increased risk of **clotting events**, such as strokes and heart attacks. When women who smoke cigarettes take OCPs containing **estrogen**, the combined effect of smoking tobacco and estrogen can further increase the risk of clot formation and related cardiovascular complications.

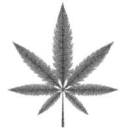

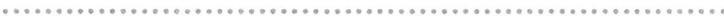

The Potential Interaction Of Cannabis Smoke And OCPs

While specific studies on the combination of smoking cannabis and taking OCPs are limited, it's reasonable to consider that similar principles may apply. Cannabis smoke, like tobacco smoke, contains numerous chemicals that can have various effects on your cardiovascular system. Additionally, smoking, in general, is associated with increased risks of cardiovascular problems. Therefore, it's advisable for women who smoke cannabis and are considering or using OCPs to consult their healthcare provider for personalized advice and guidance based on their specific situation. This's especially relevant for women who are already at a higher risk due to factors such as age, obesity, or a personal or family history of cardiovascular diseases.

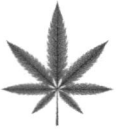

The potential risks associated with smoking cannabis while using OCPs should not be taken lightly. Women should be aware that the combined effect of these two factors can further elevate the risk of blood clot formation and related adverse events.

46

It's important to note that the relationship between smoking, homocysteine levels, and clot formation is complex and multifactorial. While smoking can contribute to increased homocysteine levels, it's not the sole determinant. Other factors, such as dietary factors and **genetic predisposition**, also play a role in homocysteine metabolism. More on the relationship between smoking and homocysteine later.

Unravelling The Context Behind Asthma Relief From Cannabis Smoke

Some people have found relief from **asthma** symptoms by smoking cannabis. Individual experiences are typically tricky to generalize. These anecdotes should be taken with a grain of salt. This's because they can result from anything from a genuine effect to the simple illusion of needing something to work to alleviate medical symptoms. One of the problems is that these people proceed to proclaim their newfound wisdom from the relief they got from the miracle plant.

Now, this's dangerous whether or not these people are right about cannabis helping with asthma symptoms. Suppose the reported impact is nothing more than a misguided belief. In that case, there's a risk that people who use cannabis will use it as a desperate plea to relieve their asthma symptoms. On the other hand, if these anecdotes are correct, then there's also a risk of overconsumption of cannabis that may lead to its own problems. It's not uncommon for some people to think that if one works, ten must work even better. There's a significant chance that these individuals will exponentially increase their vulnerability to the complications of cannabis consumption.

It's crucial to approach individual anecdotes cautiously and not generalize their experiences to the broader population. While valuable from particular perspectives, anecdotal evidence doesn't provide conclusive scientific evidence of efficacy or safety.

47

Asthma is a complex condition, and its management typically involves evidence-based medical treatments, such as **bronchodilators** and anti-inflammatory medications. While some individuals may report finding relief from asthma symptoms through cannabis use, it's crucial to note that the effects of cannabis can vary from person to person, and what works for one individual may not work for another.

Furthermore, self-medicating with cannabis for asthma without proper medical guidance can be risky. Cannabis contains various compounds, including THC and CBD, which can affect your respiratory system and overall health differently. Overconsumption or misuse of cannabis can lead to potential adverse effects, such as **respiratory irritation**, increased heart rate, **cognitive impairment**, and dependency.

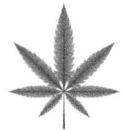

The scientific research on the direct link between cannabis use and asthma is limited, and further studies are needed to understand the potential effects fully. It's crucial to rely on evidence-based research when making conclusions about the relationship between cannabis and asthma.

While it's known that some asthma triggers can be psychological, such as stress and anxiety, it's essential to note that asthma is a complex respiratory condition with multiple factors contributing to its development and symptoms. Asthma involves chronic inflammation and constriction of the airways, leading to breathing difficulties and asthma attacks.

While cannabis may have some relaxing effects and potentially help with stress and anxiety, the specific impact of cannabis on asthma symptoms is not well-established. In fact, smoking cannabis can introduce irritants and potentially harmful substances into your respiratory system, which could exacerbate asthma symptoms and pose risks to your lung health.

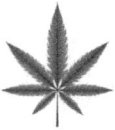

48

As more research is conducted on the potential effects of cannabis on asthma, a more precise understanding may emerge. However, until then, individuals with asthma should prioritize proven medical treatments and consult with healthcare professionals for personalized care.

The limited research on the use of cannabis for asthma suggests potential mixed effects, and it's essential to consider both the potential benefits and risks. While some studies indicate that certain components of cannabis may have anti-inflammatory properties that could help reduce airway inflammation in asthma, more research is needed to fully understand the specific mechanisms and overall efficacy.

However, it's important to note that smoking, whether cannabis or any other substance, can introduce irritants and potentially harmful substances into your respiratory system. Smoke inhalation, including second hand smoke, can trigger asthma symptoms and worsen asthma attacks in susceptible individuals. This applies to cannabis smoke as well.

Inhaling smoke, regardless of the source, can irritate your airways, leading to **bronchial constriction** and increased mucus production, which are hallmark features of asthma. Therefore, it's generally recommended for individuals with asthma to avoid smoking, including cannabis, to reduce the risk of exacerbating their symptoms.

Ultimately, the decision to use cannabis for asthma should be made in consultation with healthcare professionals who can provide personalized guidance based on your specific condition, medical history, and available evidence. Prioritizing proven medical treatments and minimizing potential risks to your respiratory health is vital.

It's also possible to develop any of the **Chronic Obstructive Pulmonary Diseases** (COPDs) like Chronic Bronchitis, **Emphysema**, **Refractory** (non-reversible) **asthma**, **Bronchiectasis**, and **Chronic Bronchiolitis** if you smoke cannabis in excess. However, the "excess" amount hasn't been addressed or defined as of the publication of this book. COPD is currently in North America's top five leading causes of death, and widespread unregulated cannabis use may not help reduce fatality.

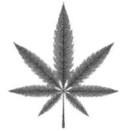

49

Once upon a time, there was a fellow who decided to trade-in his solid conservative upbringing for a taste of the ultra-liberal life. Oh boy, did he get more than he bargained for! He was lured by the allure of excitement and something completely different, but little did he know that it would consume him like a kid in a candy store.
In this brave new world, everything was topsy-turvy and unfamiliar. It was like he had landed on an alien planet with its own rules and customs. Poor chap, he struggled to adapt and fit in. It was like trying to wear shoes that were three sizes too small. Ouch!

Looking back, you can't help but wonder if he should have taken things a bit more slowly. Baby steps, my friend! Start with dipping a toe in the water instead of doing a cannonball into the deep end. Maybe he needed a trusty guide who could show him the ropes and help him find his place in this wild and crazy society. But alas, he didn't seek a guru's wisdom; instead, he dove headfirst into a whirlwind of chaos.

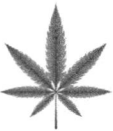

50

Change, my friends, is no walk in the park. It's like trying to solve a Rubik's Cube with your eyes closed while riding a unicycle. Everyone has their own tolerance for change and unique way of handling it. Unfortunately, our protagonist's thirst for novelty and adventure led him down a treacherous path. It's a stark reminder that we must choose our paths wisely and be aware of the consequences they may bring.

So, my fellow adventurers, let this cautionary tale be a reminder that change can be a tricky beast. It's like a roller coaster ride with unexpected twists and turns. Take a moment to think before you make that leap. Seek guidance if needed. And always keep in mind that life is a series of choices, and it's up to us to navigate the crazy maze of possibilities. May your choices lead you to beautiful adventures and not down a rabbit hole of regrets!

When You Know, You Know

What Are Epithelial Cells?

Let's embark on a fascinating journey through the wondrous world of your body's protective lining, the **epithelial cells**! Picture this: inside your body, every tissue and organ is like a bustling city with its own unique environment, and these epithelial cells are like the trusty guardians that line the streets and protect the buildings.

Now, these epithelial cells are a diverse bunch. Like superheroes have different powers to match their challenges, epithelial cells in various organs have unique features to tackle the specific demands of their respective environments. It's like having a team of specialized defenders ready to take on any threat!

Take a look at your blood vessels, for instance. These highways of your circulatory system transport blood throughout your body, ensuring oxygen and nutrients reach every nook and cranny. But with all that blood rushing through, blood vessels face a fair share of abrasion. To deal with this constant friction, the epithelial cells lining your blood vessels have a unique structure that makes them tough and resilient, like a superhero wearing an armour suit. They're designed to withstand the forces of flowing blood, keeping your blood vessels intact and preventing any leaks or damage.

Now, let's make a detour to your stomach, where a completely different scene unfolds. Your stomach, my friend, is a powerhouse of digestion. It churns and mixes food with a mighty force. But here's the twist: your stomach secretes a highly corrosive substance called **hydrochloric acid** to break down food and kick-start digestion. It's like a volcano of acidity, ready to dissolve anything in its path.

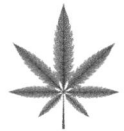

51

Enter the specialized epithelial cells lining your stomach. They're the ultimate defenders against the acid onslaught. These incredible cells produce a thick mucus layer that coats your stomach lining, acting as a shield against the corrosive effects of hydrochloric acid. It's like they're wearing a superhero cape made of mucus, protecting the delicate stomach tissues from harm. Without this protective mucus layer, the acid would wreak havoc, causing discomfort, **nausea**, and hindering proper digestion.

The columnar epithelial cells lining your bronchioles, those tiny airways in your lungs, have some pretty cool superpowers. They possess the ability to secrete chemicals that can **detoxify** certain toxins that you may inhale. Think of them as your body's defence team, working tirelessly to neutralize harmful substances and protect your respiratory system.

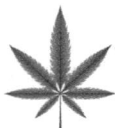

52

Now, when it comes to your skin, another group of remarkable epithelial cells comes into play. These are called **squamous epithelial** cells. They're found in areas of your body that experience high levels of abrasion, such as the outer layer of your skin. Picture them as the formidable warriors guarding the frontlines, facing constant rubbing, friction, and exposure to the elements.

Interestingly, the type of epithelial cells present in a particular tissue or organ depends on that environment's specific demands and challenges. Epithelial cells are like adaptable superheroes, capable of changing their characteristics to cope with new conditions. When the environment of a tissue changes, these cells have the remarkable ability to adjust and adapt their structure and function to ensure the ongoing protection of that tissue.

For example, suppose a tissue is exposed to increased stress or introduces a new stressor. In that case, the epithelial cells may undergo changes to handle the situation better. This adaptation helps to maintain the integrity and functionality of the tissue, preventing organ damage and promoting overall health.

Suppose the epithelial cells fail to adapt adequately to the new stressor or environmental change. In that case, the tissue may become vulnerable to damage. This can affect the tissue's structure and function, leading to potential health issues.

Understanding the importance of these adaptable epithelial cells highlights the significance of their role in protecting our bodies. They're a vital component of our defence mechanisms, helping to safeguard tissues and organs from various stressors and maintaining their proper function.

What Is Metaplasia?

When tissues are exposed to new environments or stressors, their epithelial cells can transform from one type to another, and this process is called **metaplasia**. Metaplasia is an evident sign of cellular changes and can occur in various tissues throughout your body. However, it's essential to closely monitor metaplasia because if it persists or progresses, it can lead to **dysplasia**. Dysplasia involves cells' abnormal growth and development, which can be a precursor to **cancer**.

53

Let's take the example of respiratory epithelium metaplasia. The respiratory system is lined with specialized **columnar epithelial cells**, which are well-suited for their role in protecting the airways. However, when exposed to certain irritants or **chronic inflammation**, the respiratory epithelium may undergo metaplasia and transform into squamous epithelial cells.

The presence of squamous cells in respiratory secretions, such as **phlegm** or **sputum**, could indicate potential issues, including **lung cancer**. Coughing up phlegm-containing squamous cells may prompt fur-

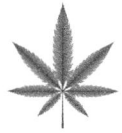

ther investigation to rule out any underlying problems and ensure timely intervention.

Monitoring metaplasia is comparable to performing routine maintenance on a car engine. Just as regular oil changes help identify and address any issues before they escalate, regular monitoring of metaplasia allows healthcare professionals to detect any cellular changes early on. This proactive approach enables timely interventions and can help prevent the progression of potentially harmful conditions.

What Is Dysplasia?

When epithelial cells undergo metaplasia, there is a risk that the new cells may become disorganized and arranged haphazardly over time as the cells naturally turn over. It's crucial to note that while metaplasia itself is reversible, meaning the cells can revert to their original form once the underlying stressor is removed, dysplasia is typically irreversible. Dysplasia refers to the abnormal growth and development of cells, and it often manifests as disorganized and structurally altered tissue.

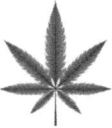

54

In cases of dysplasia, the cells may lose their normal attachment to each other, leading to a lack of proper tissue structure and function. This disorganization and loss of normal cell structure can be an early indication of potential problems, including an increased risk of developing cancer.
The progression from metaplasia to dysplasia and potentially to cancer underscores the importance of minimizing or avoiding changes in the environment of epithelial cells within a specific tissue. Persistent irritation or exposure to certain risk factors can contribute to metaplasia, which, if left unchecked, may progress to dysplasia before eventually developing into cancer.

You can focus on preventive measures and interventions to mitigate the risk factors associated with cellular changes by understanding the relationship between metaplasia, dysplasia, and cancer. This highlights the significance of early detection, prompt medical attention, and the implementation of strategies to reduce or eliminate exposure to irritants or risk factors known to induce metaplasia.

Maintaining a healthy lifestyle, avoiding known **carcinogens**, and undergoing regular screenings and check-ups can contribute to overall wellness and potentially prevent the development of cancers rooted in metaplasia and subsequent dysplasia.

How Do Your Lungs Protect You From The Undesirables You Inhale?

It's fascinating how your lungs are naturally equipped to handle pure gases like oxygen and carbon dioxide. However, when toxic gases are introduced into your respiratory system, they can irritate and trigger changes in the **lung architecture**.

The columnar epithelial cells in your bronchioles secrete substances that help detoxify and counteract harmful agents you breathe in, which include **vitamin C**.
Vitamin C acts as an **antioxidant** in your body. Antioxidants are substances that help neutralize harmful **free radicals** and **oxidative stress**. Free radicals are unstable molecules that can cause damage to your cells, including your **DNA**, if their levels become excessive or prolonged. This oxidative stress can contribute to the development of various health conditions, including cancer.

By acting as an antioxidant, vitamin C helps neutralize the harmful effects of free radicals and other toxins in your respiratory system. This protective mechanism is an important defence mechanism of your lungs to maintain their health and integrity.

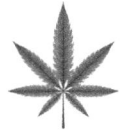

55

When you inhale cigarette or cannabis smoke, it can irritate the columnar epithelial cells that line your bronchioles. This irritation is a result of the toxic components present in the smoke. Over time, chronic exposure to smoke and the resulting irritation can lead to changes in the environment of your bronchioles. In response to this persistent irritation, the columnar epithelial cells may transform into squamous epithelial cells, also called **squamous metaplasia**.

The transformation from columnar to squamous epithelial cells is considered a protective mechanism. Squamous epithelial cells can better withstand the ongoing irritation caused by smoke. Dysplasia can then occur as a result of prolonged exposure to smoke and the associated metaplasia. If left unchecked, this can progress to the development of **squamous cell carcinoma**, a type of lung cancer.

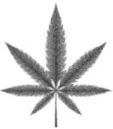

Why Do People Differ In Their Susceptibility To Lung Damage From Smoke?

56

People differ in their susceptibility to the harmful effects of smoke exposure due to a combination of factors such as diet, physiology, genetics, and environmental influences. While it's generally true that prolonged exposure to smoke increases the risk of developing lung cancer, there're individual variations in the tolerance to stressors. Some individuals may have a lower threshold for the detrimental effects of smoke, which can lead to cancer development at an earlier stage than others.

Genetics also plays a significant role in lung cancer susceptibility. Certain genetic variations and defects can increase the risk of developing lung diseases, including lung cancer. These genetic factors can range from minor variations to more significant inherited mutations, which can impact your predisposition to developing cancer.

It's important to note that there're different types of lung cancer, each with distinct causes and disease progressions. The type of cancer discussed here, Squamous Cell Carcinoma, refers explicitly to the epithelial cells in your lungs that undergo metaplasia and transform from columnar to squamous. This type of lung cancer is named after the specific cell type involved and its cancerous growth.

What's The Difference In Lung Damage Between Cigarettes And Cannabis?

Cigarettes have been extensively studied, and their specific chemicals have been found to have detrimental effects on lung cells, leading to certain types of cancer. However, the research on the long-term effects of cannabis smoking is still relatively limited compared to cigarettes.

Cannabis smoke contains many of the same harmful chemicals as tobacco smoke, including carcinogens such as **benzene**, **formaldehyde**, and **polycyclic aromatic hydrocarbons** (PAHs). These chemicals have been associated with cellular changes and an increased risk of cancer development.

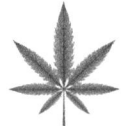

57

The direct relationship between smoke irritation and the development of Squamous Cell Carcinoma is observed in both cigarette smoking and cannabis smoking. Squamous Cell Carcinoma is currently the most common type of lung cancer in male smokers, highlighting the harmful impact of smoke on lung tissue.

It's important to note that while Squamous Cell Carcinoma is more commonly associated with smoke irritation, other types of lung cancer can also result from cannabis smoking, albeit indirectly. For example, **adenocarcinoma** of the lungs, which is the most common type of lung cancer in nonsmokers and female smokers, can also occur due to long-term cannabis smoking. The mechanisms by which cannabis smoke may contribute to the development of different types of lung cancer are still being investigated.

What's The Relationship Between Glaucoma And Cannabis?

Cannabis has various strains and contains different active ingredients, which can result in different effects on your body. While some effects of cannabis are well-known, there're still areas where further research is needed to fully understand its potential benefits and risks.

One example where cannabis has shown potential benefits is in relieving the symptoms of **glaucoma**. This eye condition can lead to blindness. Glaucoma encompasses a group of eye diseases characterized by damage to the **optic nerve**, a nerve responsible for transmitting visual information from your eye to your brain. This damage is often associated with **increased intraocular pressure** (IOP), the pressure inside your eye. IOP can exert compression on the delicate fibres of your optic nerve, leading to vision loss over time.

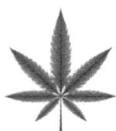

58

Cannabis, precisely its active compounds, has been found to have the ability to lower IOP. This effect is thought to be mediated by activating cannabinoid receptors in your eyes, which helps regulate fluid flow and drainage in your eye, thereby reducing IOP. By lowering IOP, cannabis may provide temporary relief for individuals with glaucoma and potentially slow the progression of the disease.

However, it's important to note that using cannabis as a treatment for glaucoma isn't without limitations. The effects are typically short-lived, requiring frequent administration, and the long-term efficacy and safety of cannabis for glaucoma management are still under investigation. Additionally, the psychoactive effects of cannabis and individual variations in response to this treatment may also need to be considered.

What are tears, and what is their purpose?

Tears are a remarkable and multi-functional fluid that contributes to your eyes' overall health and well-being. They are composed of a combination of water, oils, mucus, **enzymes**, **antibodies**, and other substances. Here are some key roles that tears play in maintaining the health and function of your eyes:

- **Lubrication:** Tears act as a natural lubricant, keeping the surface of your eye moist and ensuring smooth movement of the eyelids and eyelashes. This lubrication is crucial for comfortable vision and preventing the sensation of dryness or irritation.
- **Cleaning:** Tears contain enzymes and antibodies that help cleanse your eye's surface by removing debris, dust, and bacteria. They flush away foreign particles that may enter your eyes, reducing the risk of infections and maintaining a clear visual pathway.
- **Nutrition:** Tears provide essential nutrients, oxygen, and other beneficial substances to your eyes' surface. These nutrients support the nourishment and health of your eyes' tissues, including your cornea, which is responsible for transmitting and focusing light.
- **Protection:** Tears create a protective barrier that shields your eyes from potential harm. They help to wash away irritants, such as dust or allergens, reducing the risk of eye irritation or injury. Additionally, the oil component of tears helps prevent evaporation and maintain a stable tear film on your eye's surface.
- **Emotional response:** Tears are closely linked to your emotional reactions. Crying is a natural way for your body to express emotions like sadness, happiness, or even frustration. Emotional tears contain additional chemicals and hormones re leased during heightened emotions, potentially providing a cathartic and stress-relieving effect.

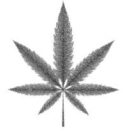

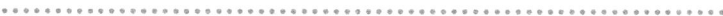

59

Overall, tears are a complex mixture that performs a range of functions to protect, nourish, and maintain the health of your eyes. However, suppose you frequently experience dryness, irritation, or other persistent eye-related concerns. In that case, it's advisable to consult an eye care professional for a comprehensive evaluation and appropriate management.

What is glaucoma?

Open-angle glaucoma, specifically **primary open-angle glaucoma** (POAG), is a progressive eye condition that develops gradually over time. It's often referred to as the "silent thief of sight" because it typically doesn't cause noticeable symptoms in its early stages.

In open-angle glaucoma, IOP gradually increases due to an imbalance between the production of **aqueous humour** and its drainage. Aqueous humour is a special kind of tears that is found within your eyes. You can wipe down excessive tear production, but aqueous humour can only accumulate in your eyes, resulting in intense eye pain.

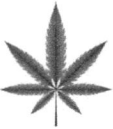

60

Excessive aqueous humour production, combined with normal drainage, can contribute to increased IOP. However, it's important to note that tears and the drainage of tears through the lacrimal ducts aren't directly related to the development or progression of glaucoma. The drainage of tears into your nasal cavity is a separate physiological process. Yes, tears drain into your nasal cavity, which is why you feel running down your nose when you're crying.

As the IOP rises over time, it can lead to damage to your optic nerve. This damage initially affects your **peripheral vision**, and as the disease progresses, it can gradually lead to the loss of **central vision**. It's like the story of the frog in boiling water: gradually increasing temperatures never cross the threshold necessary for the frog to realize its danger until it's too late to jump out.

The gradual nature of open-angle glaucoma makes it challenging to detect and diagnose in its early stages. Many individuals may only realize they have the condition once they undergo a comprehensive eye examination or experience significant vision loss. That's why regular eye examinations are crucial for early detection and treatment, especially for individuals at higher risk (such as those with a family history of glaucoma or older adults).

Angle-closure glaucoma, whether acute or chronic, is a condition where aqueous humour drainage from your eyes is impaired, leading to increased IOP. This increased pressure can cause rapid and severe damage to your optic nerve, leading to vision loss or blindness if not promptly treated.

In angle-closure glaucoma, the drainage angle between your cornea and **iris** becomes narrow or completely blocked, preventing your eye's normal outflow of aqueous humour. Angle-closure glaucoma is like a clogged drain pipe -- the fluid that should be flowing away gets stuck and builds up, causing pressure to increase and eventually causing severe damage if not addressed.

61

Acute angle-closure glaucoma is characterized by a sudden and severe increase in IOP, causing intense eye pain, **blurred vision**, **halos** around lights, and sometimes nausea and vomiting. This's a medical emergency that requires immediate attention to relieve the pressure and prevent further damage to your optic nerve.

Chronic angle-closure glaucoma, on the other hand, develops gradually over time with intermittent or mild symptoms. It may not present with the same acute symptoms as the sudden form, but it still requires proper management and treatment to prevent vision loss in the long run.
Both forms of angle-closure glaucoma can cause irreversible damage to your optic nerve if left untreated.

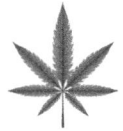

Therefore, seeking immediate medical attention is crucial if you experience any sudden onset of severe eye pain, visual disturbances, or other concerning symptoms.

Treatment for angle-closure glaucoma typically involves lowering your IOP through medication, laser procedures, or surgery to create a new drainage pathway for aqueous humour to leave your eyes. The specific treatment approach will depend on the severity and underlying cause of the condition.

How does cannabis help relieve symptoms of glaucoma?

Cannabis has shown potential therapeutic effects in reducing IOP in individuals with glaucoma. Studies have indicated that the active compounds in cannabis, mainly THC and CBD, can decrease IOP by enhancing the outflow of aqueous humour from your eyes. By increasing the outflow of aqueous humour, the pressure inside your eyes can be reduced.

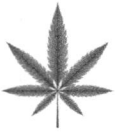

62

When THC and CBD stimulate cannabinoid receptors, it leads to the relaxation of the **ciliary muscle**. The ciliary muscle is a ring-shaped muscle located in your eyes. When it contracts or relaxes, it controls the shape of your **lens**, which is essential for focusing on objects at different distances. When THC and CBD stimulate the cannabinoid receptors in your eyes, the **ciliary muscle** tends to relax.

THC and CBD can also relax the opening of the **trabecular meshwork**. The trabecular meshwork is a mesh-like tissue near your eyes' front. It acts as a drainage pathway for aqueous humour. The aqueous humour can drain out of your eyes when the trabecular meshwork is open. This enhanced outflow helps to lower your IOP.

In addition to its potential IOP-lowering effects, cannabis may also have **neuroprotective** properties that could be beneficial in glaucoma. Studies have suggested that cannabinoids may help protect your optic nerve from damage and slow down the progression of the disease. However, more research is needed to fully understand the extent and mechanisms of these neuroprotective effects.

It's important to note that while cannabis may provide temporary relief by reducing IOP, it shouldn't be considered a standalone treatment for glaucoma. Traditional treatments, such as eye drops and medications, are typically the primary methods for managing glaucoma and preventing vision loss. These treatments are specifically tailored to target IOP and have been extensively studied and proven effective.

What's The Relationship Between Cannabis And Stimulating Appetite?

Cannabis has been found to effectively increase appetite and reduce nausea, making it valuable in managing symptoms and improving the quality of life for some chronically ill patients. The phenomenon of increased appetite, commonly known as "the munchies," is a well-known side effect of cannabis use. When cannabis is consumed, particularly strains high in THC, it can enhance the desire for food and promote hunger. Recognizing this effect, researchers explored the potential of cannabis in addressing appetite loss and weight loss experienced by patients with conditions like cancer, HIV/AIDS, or other chronic illnesses.

To harness the appetite-stimulating properties of cannabis while minimizing the risks associated with smoking, pharmaceutical companies focused on isolating specific active chemicals found in cannabis. One of these chemicals is CBD, which has gained attention for its therapeutic potential without causing the intoxicating effects associated with THC.

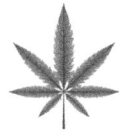

Pharmaceutical companies developed CBD-based medications that specifically target appetite stimulation and nausea suppression. By isolating and formulating CBD into pills or other controlled dosage forms, patients can experience the benefits without exposure to potentially harmful smoke or unwanted psychoactive effects.

Utilizing a known drug's side effect for a different medical purpose is not uncommon in medicine. Drugs such as those for **erectile dysfunction** emerged from similar observations and research. By identifying the active chemical responsible for a particular effect, scientists can develop medications that provide targeted benefits while minimizing potential risks.

It's important to note that using CBD or cannabis-derived medications for appetite stimulation should be done under the guidance of healthcare professionals. They can assess your specific medical needs, consider potential drug interactions, and determine the most appropriate dosage and administration method.

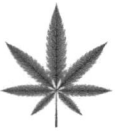

64

The evolving understanding of cannabis and its potential medical applications has led to a shift in perception and acceptance in recent years. While cannabis was once stigmatized and demonized, research and clinical evidence have demonstrated its therapeutic value in addressing various diseases and symptoms.

By exploring and isolating specific compounds found in cannabis, such as THC and CBD, scientists and pharmaceutical companies have been able to develop medications that provide targeted benefits while minimizing unwanted effects. This approach allows for more precise and controlled use of the plant's properties.

The potential of cannabis as a medical tool is vast, and ongoing research continues to uncover new applications and benefits. It has shown promise in managing pain, reducing inflammation, alleviating symptoms of neurological disorders, treating **epilepsy**, and more. Additionally, several countries have approved cannabis-based medications for specific medical conditions.

While the medical use of cannabis is becoming increasingly recognized, it's essential to note that further research is needed to understand its potential benefits and risks fully. Regulations and guidelines are in place to ensure safe and appropriate use, and healthcare professionals play a crucial role in guiding patients toward evidence-based treatments.

As scientific knowledge expands and more research is conducted, the therapeutic potential of cannabis may continue to grow, offering new avenues for treating and managing various diseases.

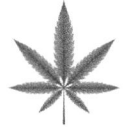

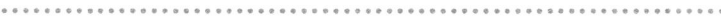

Understanding the complexities of human behaviour, especially in the context of minors experiencing stress, is indeed a challenge. It's essential to approach these issues with empathy, compassion, and a willingness to delve deeper into the underlying causes rather than merely focusing on the outward manifestations.

The manifestations of stress or emotional struggles in minors can vary widely, and it's crucial to recognize that these behaviours are often symptoms of deeper underlying issues. By addressing the root causes, we can provide appropriate support and interventions to help individuals navigate their challenges and promote their well-being.

It is essential to move away from stigmatizing or labelling individuals based solely on their outward behaviours. Efforts should be focused on understanding the unique circumstances and contexts in which these behaviours arise. Factors such as family dynamics, social environment, cultural background, economic circumstances, and personal experiences can all manifest stress or mental health difficulties.

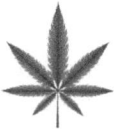

66

Taking a comprehensive approach to mental health involves considering various factors that may contribute to a person's well-being. This includes addressing financial stress, fostering healthy relationships, promoting social connectedness, and providing resources for support and coping strategies.

We can develop more targeted and effective interventions by prioritizing, identifying, and understanding the root causes of social problems. This requires collaborative efforts involving parents, educators, mental health professionals, and the community at large.

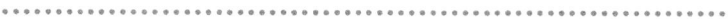

An earthquake can destroy an entire country, but it first hits only one point on the earth's surface, the epicentre, before spreading. This epicentre would have originated deep in the earth at a point called the focus. The root of a social problem is like the focus of an earthquake.

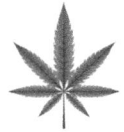

67

Getting in is Easy, But Staying in is Messy

Your Body: From Cell to Organism

In the fascinating world of biology, understanding the workings of our bodies starts at the tiniest building blocks called **cells**. A group of cells of the same type is called a **tissue**, which in turn combines with other tissues of the same type to form an **organ**. Finally, organs link up with other organs to form an **organism**. Like how individual LEGO bricks combine to create a magnificent castle, cells team up to construct the complex machinery of our bodies.

What we observe on or in an organism—whether as an effect of medication, normal body processes, or even a lack of response—all starts at the cellular level. It's undoubtedly the micro that makes up the macro. It's like playing detective to uncover the hidden secrets behind the observed effects. You see, cells are remarkable entities with specialized functions. Different types of cells form various tissues, such as muscle, nerve, or epithelial tissues, each with a unique role in your body's grand symphony.

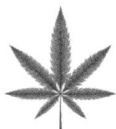

68

A small effect on cells can be seen as anything from diarrhea and muscle twitching to abnormal heart rhythms and **seizures**. When we talk about the effects of cannabis on the general population, a scientist can only wonder what might be happening at the cellular level, which could result in the observed effects.

Analyzing the Effect of Cannabis at the Cellular Level

Cannabis contains active compounds like THC and CBD that interact with your cells in intriguing ways. These compounds can bind to specific receptors found on the surface of cells, just like a key fitting into a lock. This interaction sets off a cascade of events within your cells, influencing their behaviour and potentially triggering a chain reaction in the surrounding tissues and organs.

For instance, when THC engages with your brain cells, it can affect your perception, mood, and even alter your sensory experiences. On the other hand, CBD might interact with cells in your immune system, influencing inflammation or immune responses. These cellular interactions are like intricate dances, with cannabis compounds guiding the steps.

Understanding the cellular effects of cannabis is a complex task, as it involves studying how these compounds interact with specific cell receptors, influence **signalling pathways**, and impact the overall function of tissues and organs. Scientists employ various research techniques, including laboratory studies, animal models, and even clinical trials involving human participants, to unravel the mysteries of cellular interactions.

By delving into the cellular realm, researchers can gain insights into how cannabis affects your body, both in beneficial and potentially harmful ways. This knowledge helps healthcare professionals make informed decisions and recommendations, ensuring the safe and effective use of cannabis-based treatments.

Cannabis has been reported to have various effects on individuals, ranging from pain relief to improvements in seizure control and psychiatric symptoms like anxiety. While these anecdotal accounts are intriguing, it's vital to approach them with caution due to the limited scientific research available on the physiological effects of cannabis.

To shed light on this subject, we can use our existing knowledge of the human body and draw parallels with the interactions of cannabis and other drugs. By doing so, we can gain some insights into how cannabis might

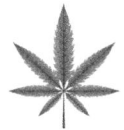

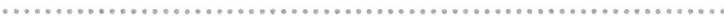

69

potentially affect normal human body processes.

For example, your body has a complex system called the **endocannabinoid system** (ECS), which plays a role in regulating various physiological processes such as pain, mood, appetite, and inflammation. Cannabis contains compounds that can interact with this system, potentially influencing its activity and subsequently affecting these processes.

Furthermore, we can examine how other medications or substances with similar properties to cannabis interact with our bodies. For instance, some pain medications, like **opioids**, can bind to brain and **spinal cord** receptors to alleviate pain. Similarly, cannabinoids in cannabis might interact with specific receptors to modulate pain perception.

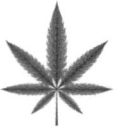

Additionally, some anti-seizure medications work by stabilizing abnormal electrical activity in your brain. It's possible that certain compounds in cannabis could also have an impact on neuronal activity, potentially explaining reports of seizure reduction in some individuals.

70

Regarding psychiatric disorders, different medications target specific neurotransmitters in your brain to modulate mood and alleviate symptoms. Although the effects of cannabis on psychiatric conditions are not yet fully understood, it's plausible that certain compounds in cannabis might interact with neurotransmitter systems, potentially providing relief for some individuals.

While this approach of extrapolating from existing knowledge can provide some insight into the potential effects of cannabis, it's crucial to emphasize the need for robust scientific research to validate these claims. Rigorous studies, including clinical trials, are necessary to establish the safety, efficacy, and appropriate use of cannabis-based treatments for various conditions.

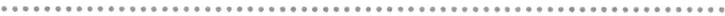

Understanding the impact of cannabis on the human body processes is crucial for effectively dealing with both cannabis use and cannabis abuse. While our general body processes are similar, individual variations can cause different responses to the same drug.

To ensure proper diagnosis and treatment of cannabis-related issues, it's essential to comprehend how cannabis affects various physiological processes. This knowledge allows healthcare professionals to make informed decisions and provide appropriate care.

It's estimated that around 3 in 10 individuals who use marijuana may develop a marijuana use disorder, indicating the potential for dependency or addiction. Moreover, there is a 10% risk of addiction for those who use cannabis. It's essential to recognize that while cannabis can have beneficial and therapeutic effects when used appropriately, excessive or irresponsible use can lead to dangerous and potentially life-threatening consequences.

Understanding Cellular Physiology in Relation to Cannabis Effects

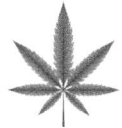

71

Before a cell can do its work, it must be activated, and this process is known as **depolarization**. In many cells, sodium is involved in the process of depolarization. Interestingly, cannabis may potentially interfere with this process by blocking sodium from entering cells. By blocking sodium, cannabis can make cells less active.

The implications of decreased cell activity caused by cannabis can be positive and negative. On the positive side, it can contribute to pain reduction and lower seizure activity, providing relief for individuals experiencing these conditions. However, it can also result in **sedation**, s**lower reflexes**, and **impaired motor coordination**.
To understand these effects, we can imagine the im-

pact of cannabis on your body as similar to a dimmer switch controlling the brightness of a light bulb. Just as the dimmer switch reduces the intensity of the electrical current entering the bulb, cannabis decreases the intensity of signals entering cells. This decrease in signal intensity can have a wide range of effects throughout your body, leading to both beneficial and adverse outcomes.

Cannabis use can lead to various effects on your body, many of which involve decreased activity in different tissues and systems. Some of the well-known symptoms of cannabis intoxication include:

- Dry mouth: Cannabis can reduce saliva production, leading to a dry and sticky feeling in your mouth.
- Bloodshot eyes: Using cannabis can cause blood vessels in your eyes to expand, resulting in redness and a bloodshot appearance.
- Increased appetite: Cannabis use is associated with increased food cravings, often called "the munchies."
- Altered sense of time: Users may perceive time differently, with minutes feeling like hours or vice versa.
- Impaired memory and concentration: Cannabis can affect cognitive function, making remembering information and concentrating on tasks difficult.
- Altered mood: Cannabis can induce mood changes, ranging from relaxation and euphoria to anxiety or even paranoia in some individuals.

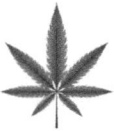

72

It's important to note that the specific symptoms and their intensity can vary from person to person. Factors such as the individual's tolerance, the strain and potency of the cannabis, and the method of consumption can all influence the effects experienced.

Some of the Proven Therapeutic Benefits of Cannabis

Research has shown promising results in using cannabis to treat diseases characterized by over-activity in cells, such as seizures, pain, and anxiety. Additionally, cannabis has been suggested to have anti-inflammatory properties and the ability to improve sleep quality.

To understand how cannabis can affect cell activity, it's helpful to consider the role of sodium and chloride ions in cellular processes. Blocking sodium from entering cells or promoting chloride influx can reduce cell activity. This mechanism has been targeted by researchers developing pharmaceuticals, including antiepileptic drugs, as well as cannabinoids that can modulate sodium channels and increase chloride influx.

One notable example is **Epidiolex**, an FDA-approved antiepileptic drug that contains a purified form of CBD derived from cannabis. Epidiolex is specifically indicated for treating seizures associated with **Lennox-Gastaut** syndrome and **Dravet syndrome**, two rare and severe forms of epilepsy, in patients aged two years and older.

73

Some pain medications and drugs for anxiety, like **barbiturates** and **benzodiazepines**, work by either blocking sodium from entering cells or promoting chloride to enter cells. Both mechanisms have the same effect: reducing a cell's activity. Most drugs currently on the market to combat seizures, pain, and anxiety use either of these mechanisms to alleviate patient suffering.

What if this's a massive coincidence that cannabis happens to help treat the same diseases treated by drugs that play around the gates for sodium or chloride? It's possible, so we must ex-

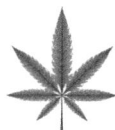

amine the **side effects** of cannabis and **anxiolytic drugs** (drugs used to treat anxiety) further.

Most drugs are designed to be specific for a particular type of receptor in your body. Since these receptors can also be found elsewhere in your body, the drug taken will end up activating all receptors of that kind throughout your body. For example, we have drugs that block **beta receptors** in your heart to slow your heart rate. These drugs are used to treat **hypertension**. However, beta receptors are also found all over your body, including other major organs like your lungs and kidneys.

When you take a beta blocker to treat hypertension, the only objective is its effect on your heart. The drug's unintended effects on other organs with beta receptors, like your lungs and kidneys, are called **side effects**. Basically, when a drug acts on a targeted receptor on a desired organ, we call that an effect. When the drug acts on the same type of receptor but on a non-desired organ, the effects are called side effects.

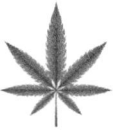

74

Side effects can vary among individuals and depend on the specific drug, dosage, individual sensitivity, and overall health status. Pharmaceutical companies strive to develop drugs with the best possible **therapeutic index** to balance desired effects and minimize unwanted side effects. The therapeutic index is a measure of a drug's safety margin that indicates the range of doses at which a drug can be used effectively while minimizing the risk of adverse effects. A high therapeutic index indicates a wide safety margin. In contrast, a low index suggests a narrower margin and higher risk of toxicity.

Possible Mechanism of Action of Cannabis in Some Organs

When cannabis acts on your brain to alleviate seizures, that is good, but it'll also work anywhere else in your body where similar receptors are found. Since our premise is that cannabis blocks sodium channels, let's see how the rest of your body would be affected. When you block sodium from entering your cells. In that case, it leads to those cells becoming less active. So, let us look at a few tissues beginning with muscles.

Muscles require **sodium influx** for proper activation and contraction. When cannabis blocks sodium channels in muscle cells, it can lead to muscle weakness. This effect can be observed in various muscles, including those controlling your eyelids, resulting in difficulty in controlling eye movements and potentially giving you a sleepy appearance. Additionally, reduced sodium influx in muscle cells can contribute to overall sluggishness and impaired reaction time, which is why cannabis can impair coordination and increase the risk of accidents when operating machinery.

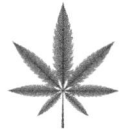

75

Moving on to the gastrointestinal system. Cannabis may have an impact on stomach movement. By reducing sodium influx into the cells of your stomach muscles, cannabis can potentially decrease the contractions and movement of your stomach. This effect may help alleviate symptoms such as a running stomach, nausea, or vomiting, relieving individuals with gastrointestinal discomfort.

Remember, the intensity of these effects can depend on factors such as the specific strain of cannabis, the dosage, and an individual's sensitivity to the drug. Additionally, the method of administration, such as smoking, vaping, or ingesting cannabis, can influence the onset and duration of these effects.

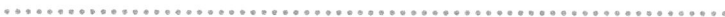

There has never been extensive research on the effects of cannabis on lowering blood pressure. Suppose the theory of blocking sodium channels holds. In that case, we may soon have a blood pressure treatment with some delightful side effects. While limited claims suggest that cannabis may lower blood pressure, more research is needed to establish a definitive link.

For the male reproductive system, things get a little complicated. In the short-term, cannabis may help achieve and sustain an **erection**, but long-term use may lead to problems getting erections. As cannabis reduces stress and anxiety, it may alleviate the blockage that prevents some men from being saluted by the one-eyed champ. However, too much cannabis can lower blood pressure too much to allow an erotic salute from the general on your command. Nearly all hypertensive medications have impotence as a side-effect, and honest cannabis users will tell you of their attempt at shooting pool with a rope.

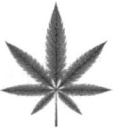

76

Another problem for men of reproductive age is trouble with **conception**. Cannabis is a **fat-soluble drug**, and its ability to cross into fat-soluble tissues, including the testes, can have implications for **sperm production** and function. Studies have suggested that cannabis use can disrupt various aspects of the reproductive process in men. Cannabis may interfere with **spermatogenesis**, which is the process of sperm production, leading to decreased sperm count, motility, and morphology. These effects can contribute to difficulties in achieving pregnancy. This's in much the same way it impacts the structure and function of neurons in your brain. A man affected by this will have a hard time firing a live round that can knock someone up.

Some research suggests that cannabis can also influence the testicles directly by inhibiting the action of **Leydig cells**. Leydig cells are specialized cells in the

testes that produce and secrete **testosterone**. They play a crucial role in male reproductive function and the development of masculine characteristics. Inhibited Leydig cells can lead to decreased testosterone production. Less testosterone means low sex drive and erectile dysfunction. In short, cannabis abuse can lead to decreased libido, impotence, and infertility.
Since cannabis affects people differently, the effects on one group are not guaranteed in another. That throws the sodium theory halfway out the window. Highly plausible, but we need to learn more. This means if this drug has so many effects and side-effects that vary across populations, it may still be in its infancy in regards to making any solid claims both for and against the drug.

Research on cannabis and its various components is ongoing, and it's still a complex and evolving field of study. While some effects of cannabis have been attributed to specific cannabinoids, other active compounds or their interactions may contribute to the observed effects. The exact mechanisms underlying the wide range of effects and side effects of cannabis are not yet fully understood.

77

To establish a clearer understanding of the effects of cannabis and its individual components, further scientific research, including well-designed clinical trials, is necessary. These studies can help unravel the complexities of cannabis and provide more evidence-based insights into its potential benefits and risks. As research progresses, our understanding of cannabis and its effects will continue to evolve, enabling more informed decisions and approaches to its use.

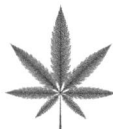

Imagine sitting by yourself in a quiet room. Time passes by, and you start to hear faint noises. You try to ignore the noises, but they only get louder. The noises come in different forms; some are more prominent than others. This gets freaky as you turn to look around but find absolutely nothing.

The noises persist. The more you try to stop the noises, the more they seem to be coming from right around you, but you still can't make sense of them. The noises keep getting louder and louder, and you feel like your ears are going to explode!

Then your friend comes in and asks why you're sitting in such a quiet room with a strange look on your face. What's the first thing that'll go through your mind after your friend asks you this? Would that make you crazy that you hear noises but your friend doesn't hear anything? What would you say back to your friend?

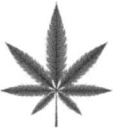

78

The most extreme silence makes the loudest noise. Inasmuch as you see with your brain, you also hear with your brain. Silence can draw attention to the finest details of any sound, both present and from memory, and your mind can accentuate or attenuate it. It's all in your mind, and when confusion ensures, you owe it to yourself to listen to an outsider to help shift your perspective.

It's Arrested Development!

While people talk a great deal about the benefits and risks of smoking cannabis, a lot has been left to the imagination for those curious about certain details about cannabis. Whether we're talking about the relaxation benefits or the risk of impairment, we still overlook some subtle but vital sub-topics that could turn this debate around for better or worse. Cannabis is most commonly known for its effects on your brain. Had this effect been absent in cannabis users, this plant would've never become as popular as it is today. Once cannabis gets into your body, what happens next?

Breaking Down Cannabis in Your Body

Once cannabis enters your body, its active compounds, such as THC and CBD, are absorbed into your bloodstream through various routes of administration, such as smoking, vaporizing, or consuming edibles. From there, the active compounds are carried to different organs and tissues throughout your body, including your brain.

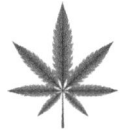

79

In your brain, cannabinoids interact with specific receptors called cannabinoid receptors, which are part of the endocannabinoid system. This system is crucial in regulating various physiological processes, including mood, appetite, pain sensation, and memory. When THC binds to cannabinoid receptors, it primarily affects the regions of the brain involved in cognition, memory, coordination, and pleasure. This interaction leads to the psychoactive and mood-altering effects commonly associated with cannabis use.

Conversely, CBD does not directly bind to cannabinoid receptors but can modulate their activity indirectly. It's believed to have a more subtle impact on your brain and may counteract some of the psychoactive effects of THC.

Apart from your brain, cannabinoids also interact with cannabinoid receptors present in other organs and tissues throughout your body. These receptors are part of the endocannabinoid system, which helps regulate various physiological functions, including immune response, inflammation, and pain perception. The specific effects of cannabis on your body depend on several factors, including the dose, method of administration, individual metabolism, and your unique endocannabinoid system. These factors contribute to the wide range of experiences and effects reported by cannabis users.

Two groups of Drugs: Fat-soluble and Water-soluble

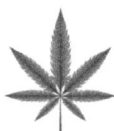

Drugs are divided into two main groups: **fat-soluble** and **water-soluble**. Fat-soluble drugs are drugs that can dissolve in fats and oils rather than in water. They can accumulate in your body's fatty tissues and remain in your body for long periods. On the other hand, water-soluble drugs are drugs that can dissolve in water rather than in fats and oils. The solubility of a drug affects its absorption, distribution, metabolism, and excretion from your body, ultimately impacting its processing and therapeutic effects.

Since fat-soluble drugs can dissolve in fats and oils, so they can easily pass through cell membranes and be absorbed into fatty tissues throughout your body. Due to their affinity for lipid-rich tissues, such as your adipose tissue, muscle, bone marrow, and brain, fat-soluble drugs can accumulate and be stored in these tissues for extended periods. This accumulation can lead to a prolonged duration of action, as the drug is slowly released back into circulation over time. However, it also means that fat-soluble drugs may take longer to be eliminated from your body.

Water-soluble drugs, on the other hand, readily dissolve in water and don't have a strong affinity for

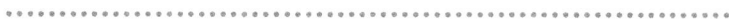

fatty tissues. They're generally absorbed more quickly into your bloodstream and distributed more evenly throughout the body's aqueous compartments. Water-soluble drugs tend to have a shorter duration of action compared to fat-soluble drugs because they're more rapidly eliminated from your body.

Since fat-soluble drugs remain in your body much longer than water-soluble drugs, this allows for extended periods of therapeutic effectiveness and adverse effects. Because of this, water-soluble drugs are usually preferred when a drug needs to be taken regularly, as they're more quickly removed from your body and pose a lower risk of building up to toxic levels in your body. This's similar to oil and water-based paints in that oil-based paints will linger on a surface for much longer and can be more challenging to remove. In contrast, water-based paints can be easily washed away with minimal effort.

Water-soluble drugs are primarily eliminated from your body through your kidneys via urine. After being absorbed into your bloodstream, water-soluble drugs undergo various processes, including metabolism and distribution to tissues. Eventually, they're filtered by your kidneys and excreted in urine.

81

Your kidneys play a crucial role in filtering waste products and drugs from your bloodstream, as well as regulating water and electrolyte balance. Your kidneys more readily filter water-soluble drugs due to their solubility in water.

Since water-soluble drugs aren't stored in fatty tissues and have a relatively shorter duration of action, they're commonly used for short-term treatments or when immediate effects are desired. Their rapid elimination from your body reduces the risk of drug accumulation or toxicity over time.

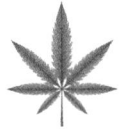

What Kind of Drug is Cannabis?

Cannabis is a fat-soluble drug, and its solubility in fats and oils allows it to dissolve in your body's fatty tissues. This occurs because the chemical constituents of cannabis, such as THC and CBD, have an affinity for fat molecules.

The structure of cell membranes consists of a **lipid bilayer** composed of **phospholipids**. These phospholipids have **hydrophilic heads** that interact with water and **hydrophobic tails** that avoid water. This arrangement forms a barrier that selectively controls the passage of substances into and out of a cell.

Since cannabis is fat-soluble, it can easily traverse cell membranes composed of lipids. Once cannabis enters your bloodstream, it can be distributed throughout your body, including fatty tissues. This distribution allows the drug to accumulate in fat cells and remain stored longer than water-soluble drugs. The fat-soluble nature of cannabis is one of the reasons it can have prolonged effects on your body. It can also be slowly released from the fatty tissues back into your bloodstream over time, contributing to its long-lasting effects.

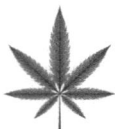

82

What's the Impact of Cannabis on the Brain?

As soon as you consume cannabis in any form, it'll leave your body and dissolve in fat-rich tissues like your muscle, **bone marrow**, brain, and even testicles. There isn't much happening in your bone marrow. However, if the effect is significant enough, cannabis can quite possibly impair some of the processes that typically occur in your bone marrow. As a drug that hasn't been extensively studied, it's too early to tell if such an association could be made with certainty. Additionally, cannabis dissolves into the **testes** (a fat-soluble drug dissolving in fatty tissue), impairing **testosterone** and **sperm** production. Of interest here for now is the effect of cannabis on your brain.

Your brain is made primarily of fat, so all fat-soluble drugs dissolve in your brain to some extent. This's not to be confused with the feeling of being high. When you're "high," the pharmacologically active form of cannabis is primarily in your blood and stimulating receptors that alter your brain chemistry. This inter-action can lead to the psychoactive and pleasurable effects commonly associated with cannabis use. How-ever, when cannabis is dissolved in your brain, it is merely there for storage.

The human brain undergoes significant development throughout childhood and adolescence, with im-portant structural and functional changes occurring during this period. Some studies suggest that regular and heavy cannabis use during this developmental stage may negatively affect brain structure, cognition, and mental health. It's been hypothesized that can-nabis use, particularly in minors, may interfere with normal brain development processes, including **syn-aptic pruning, myelination**, and **neurochemical signalling**. The endocannabinoid system is involved in these developmental processes.

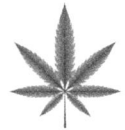

83

Synaptic pruning is a natural process in a developing brain where unnecessary or weak connections be-tween neurons are eliminated, resulting in a more refined and efficient neural network. It helps shape your brain's architecture, improve **neural circuitry**, and optimize brain function. Myelination is the pro-cess by which **axons**, the long, slender projections of neurons, are covered with a fatty substance called **myelin**. Myelin is an insulating sheath that wraps around the axon, forming a protective layer. Neuro-chemical signalling, also known as synaptic signal-ling, refers to the process by which neurons com-municate with each other through the release and reception of neurotransmitters.

The relationship between cannabis use and brain de-velopment is complex and influenced by various fac-

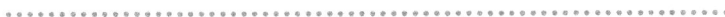

tors, including the age of onset, duration, frequency, and amount of cannabis use, as well as individual genetic and environmental factors.

It's essential to highlight that the potential risks associated with cannabis use in adolescents shouldn't be overstated. It's also crucial to consider potential **confounding factors** such as concurrent substance use and abuse, mental health conditions, and socioeconomic factors that may contribute to the observed associations.

THC has been implicated in interfering with the normal functioning of the endocannabinoid system, potentially affecting the development of brain circuits and neural pathways, particularly in regions such as your **prefrontal cortex**. Your prefrontal cortex is responsible for higher-order cognitive functions like decision-making, impulse control, and working memory. It continues to develop and mature during adolescence. Studies have suggested that regular and heavy cannabis use during this critical period may disrupt the normal development of the prefrontal cortex and impact its functional connectivity with other brain regions.

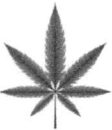

The specific mechanisms through which THC may cause brain changes and potential long-term consequences are still under investigation. It's important to note that not all young cannabis users will experience brain damage, as individual factors, including genetic predisposition, frequency and duration of use, and co-occurring environmental factors, can influence the outcomes.

While there's evidence to suggest potential risks of cannabis use on brain development, it's essential to consider the limitations of the research, such as difficulties in establishing causality and controlling for confounding factors. Additionally, it's worth noting that the effects may vary depending on individual differences and patterns of cannabis use.

Research has indicated that heavy cannabis use during adolescence is associated with certain structural and functional changes in the brain, including a reduction in brain volume in certain regions such as the **hippocampus**. The hippocampus plays a crucial role in memory and learning processes.

Longitudinal studies have demonstrated that cannabis use during adolescence is associated with lower performance on cognitive tasks assessing memory, attention, and executive functions. These effects have been observed both during periods of active cannabis use and persisting after cessation of use. Some studies suggest that cognitive deficits associated with cannabis use during adolescence may persist into adulthood.

It's important to note that the impact of cannabis on brain structure and cognitive function can be influenced by various factors, including the amount and frequency of cannabis use, the age of initiation, duration of use, and individual susceptibility. Not all individuals who use cannabis during adolescence will experience the same degree of cognitive impairments or structural changes.

85

It's worth mentioning that the brain has a certain degree of **plasticity**, and some research suggests that **cognitive deficits** associated with cannabis use may improve with abstinence and over time. However, the extent of recovery and the potential for long-term effects are still areas of active investigation.

The research on the effects of cannabis use, especially in young people, is still evolving, and there're ongoing debates and limitations in the studies conducted so far. While evidence suggests potential risks and negative impacts on brain development and cognitive function, it's essential to acknowledge that more research is needed to fully understand the extent and long-term consequences of cannabis use during adolescence.

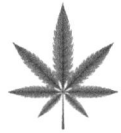

Given the vulnerabilities of the developing brain, it's generally recommended to avoid cannabis use, particularly in underage individuals. The potential risks associated with cannabis use, such as cognitive impairments and alterations in brain structure, highlight the importance of taking a cautious approach, especially during critical periods of brain development.

Cannabis Risk to the Unborn, Infants, and Toddlers

Suppose you are a minor consuming cannabis. In that case, you may suffer minor brain damage that may indirectly affect your **intellectual capacity**. Intellectual capacity refers to your ability to think, learn, understand, and reason. It can be affected by factors such as brain injury, illnesses, malnutrition, and certain drugs and toxins. Education, training, and various cognitive-enhancing activities can enhance intellectual capacity.

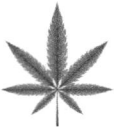

86

Some people reading this who started taking cannabis as teenagers are probably screaming at the book, claiming this to be a lie. However, observe them and learn more about their past to understand what isn't evident at first glance. However, it's worthwhile to remind you that adverse effects on intellectual capacity are not likely to be found in every single person that ever took cannabis as a teenager. The person screaming at the book might be telling the truth that cannabis never affected them. However, that only makes them an exception that proves the rule. The known fact is that many young people have suffered real and severe brain damage due to illicit drug use. You can try to fight it all you want, but that doesn't change the fact.

Let's use our imagination for a moment. If cannabis has been shown to stop or impair brain development in young adults, what do you think it will do to a toddler or an unborn child? Of course, no parent is sharing a joint with their toddler, but toddlers live in environments filled with such smoke.

Now, think about it. What are the chances of brain damage in toddlers and infants? Is there a chance they might be at a higher risk as their brains are even less developed than young adults? Should we be concerned about cannabis getting to toddlers? Is there anything we can do to stop this from happening to toddlers, at the very least? Can we think more about this? Suppose the risk of impairment to brain development and function is high in young adults and probably higher in toddlers and infants. What do you think is the level of risk to an unborn child? Of course, no one will blow smoke into an unborn child, but some will undoubtedly try. You cannot feed the fetus cannabis edibles, so how does cannabis get to the fetus? Is it possible for cannabis to cause severe and irreparable harm to the developing fetus if it gets there?

Regarding the potential effects of cannabis on toddlers, infants, and unborn children, it's essential to note that research in these specific populations is limited. A child's developing brain and body are highly sensitive to external influences, including drugs and other toxic substances. As such, it's reasonable to have concerns about the potential impact of cannabis exposure in these vulnerable stages of development.

Exposure to cannabis smoke in a toddler or infant's environment can potentially lead to inhaling secondhand smoke. This exposure may result in the absorption of certain cannabinoids, including THC, into their system. The effects of such exposure are poorly understood. They may also vary depending on factors such as the duration and intensity of exposure.

In the case of breastfeeding, THC can be transferred to the baby through breast milk if a breastfeeding mother uses cannabis. The concentration of THC in breast milk can vary depending on several factors, including

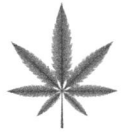

the mother's cannabis use pattern. Research suggests that THC exposure through breast milk may affect the infant's developing brain and potentially impact their **neurobehavioral development**.

Regarding the potential risks to an unborn child, it's paramount to emphasize that using cannabis during pregnancy is generally discouraged. While the **fetus** cannot directly consume cannabis as it doesn't have a direct blood supply, specific components of cannabis, including THC, can cross the **placenta** and reach the developing fetus. This exposure may potentially affect the developing brain and other organs, as well as increase the risk of complications during pregnancy.

Ultimately, more research is needed to fully understand the specific risks and long-term effects of cannabis exposure on toddlers, infants, and unborn children. In the absence of comprehensive data, it's prudent to prioritize the well-being and safety of these individuals by avoiding cannabis exposure during critical stages of development.

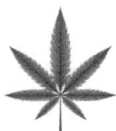

88

Minors who suffer brain damage, however mild, will have brain functions similar to someone a couple of years younger than them in terms of thinking, learning, understanding, and reasoning. It's worth mentioning that while some individuals may credit cannabis for enhancing their creativity or providing positive effects, the potential risks to brain development shouldn't be ignored or dismissed. It's essential to approach the topic with a balanced perspective, considering the potential benefits and harms.

Pregnancy, A Very Delicate Process

One of the most beautiful things in life is being able to bring another life into this world. Whether you're part of the conception or the actual event of childbirth, you deserve to feel special. The main physical job of the father to bring the unborn into the world is typically done right after conception, but it also goes into taking care of the mother-to-be throughout the process and after the child is born. Short of stressing the mother-to-be, what the father does to his body after conception doesn't affect the physical development of the unborn, but the same can't be said about the mother.

There's a vigorous debate about when life starts, which is more philosophical than scientific. One question that has never been asked in all this chaos is, "When does motherhood begin?" If being a mother is about providing for and supporting your young ones to live healthy lives, then motherhood starts long before conception. While the physical act of conception is typically attributed to the father, the role of the mother in nurturing and preparing for the well-being of her future child is profound.

Prior to conception, the mother-to-be plays a crucial role in creating a nurturing environment for the unborn child. Factors such as maintaining a healthy lifestyle, including a balanced diet, regular exercise, and avoiding harmful substances, can significantly impact the health of both the mother and the developing fetus.

During pregnancy, the mother's body undergoes remarkable changes to support the growth and development of the unborn child. The placenta, which forms within the mother's uterus, acts as a lifeline, providing essential nutrients and oxygen to the fetus while removing waste products.
The mother's choices during pregnancy, such as eating a nutritious diet, getting regular prenatal care, and avoiding harmful substances like alcohol and tobacco, directly impact the health and well-being of the developing child. These choices can influence the child's physical development, organ formation, and overall health during pregnancy and beyond.

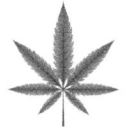

Prenatal vitamins are specifically designed to provide the necessary nutrients, such as folic acid, iron, calcium, and other essential vitamins and minerals, to support the healthy growth and development of the baby.

On the other hand, certain drugs and substances taken by pregnant women can have adverse effects on the unborn child. These substances include prescription medications, over-the-counter drugs, and recreational drugs. When pregnant women ingest these substances, these substances can cross the placenta and reach the developing fetus, potentially causing harm.

The effects of drugs during pregnancy can vary depending on the specific substance and the timing and duration of exposure. Some drugs may interfere with the normal development of organs and systems in the fetus, leading to structural abnormalities or functional impairments. Others may affect the delicate balance of neurotransmitters in the developing brain, potentially causing long-term behavioural and cognitive issues.

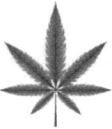

90

Learning From Past Mistakes?

Diethylstilbestrol (DES) was prescribed to pregnant women in the 1940s through the 1970s to alleviate symptoms of morning sickness and prevent miscarriages. Unfortunately, it was later discovered that DES exposure in the womb had severe long-term health consequences for the daughters of these women.

Studies conducted in the 1970s revealed a link between DES exposure and an increased risk of **clear cell carcinoma** (a type of cancer) of the **vagina** and **cervix** in the daughters of women who took DES during pregnancy. This shocking discovery led to the banning of DES in many countries and sparked awareness of the potential risks associated with prenatal drug exposure.

The daughters exposed to DES faced various health issues, including an increased risk of reproductive tract abnormalities, **infertility**, and a higher susceptibility to certain cancers. The devastating effects of DES exposure served as a powerful reminder of the importance of thorough testing and scrutiny of drugs before they are prescribed during pregnancy.

This unfortunate incident with DES prompted significant changes in medical practices and regulations. It highlighted the need for rigorous testing and monitoring of drugs for potential harmful effects on both the pregnant woman and the developing fetus. Today, extensive research and regulatory measures are in place to ensure drug safety during pregnancy.

It's important to note that DES was an extreme case, and most medications used during pregnancy undergo a thorough evaluation and are prescribed cautiously. However, this cautionary tale reminds us of the potential risks associated with prenatal drug exposure and the importance of ongoing research and monitoring to ensure the well-being of both mothers and their unborn children.

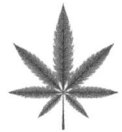

91

The Rise of Fetal Alcohol Syndrome

Fetal alcohol syndrome (FAS) has emerged as a leading cause of **intellectual impairment**, surpassing **Down syndrome** in North America. FAS is a condition that occurs when a developing fetus is exposed to alcohol during pregnancy. The harmful effects of alcohol on the developing brain can lead to a range of physical, cognitive, and behavioural impairments. They often include intellectual impairment, learning difficulties, developmental delays, behavioural problems, and physical abnormalities.

The fetus's brain development is particularly vulnerable during the early weeks of pregnancy. The formation of the brain begins around three weeks after conception. The most significant parts of brain development are completed by approximately eight weeks. During this critical period, between three and eight weeks, the brain is most susceptible to damage from alcohol exposure.

One of the common whistleblowers for a possible pregnancy is a **missed period** followed by **morning sickness**. A missed period of serious concern typically occurs about six weeks after conception. Morning sickness tends to be a symptom occurring around eight to twelve weeks after conception. Remember, when you drink while pregnant, your baby also drinks.

When a pregnant woman consumes alcohol, it enters her bloodstream and can cross the placenta, reaching the developing fetus. The fetus shares the same blood supply as the mother, which means that any alcohol consumed by the mother also affects the baby. Alcohol can disrupt the normal development of brain cells and interfere with the formation of neural connections, leading to structural and functional abnormalities in the brain.

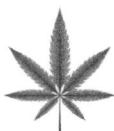

Alcohol is a water-soluble drug and primarily stays in your bloodstream. However, the **blood-brain barrier**, which helps protect your brain from potentially harmful substances in your blood, isn't fully developed before the eighth week of pregnancy. During this critical period, alcohol, due to its small size, can diffuse through the developing blood-brain barrier and reach the vulnerable brain of the fetus.

Basic principles of chemical distribution govern the distribution of alcohol throughout your body. The goal of the body's distribution system is to maintain equilibrium and distribute substances, including alcohol, to areas where they can be stored or metabolized. Unfortunately, in the case of alcohol exposure during pregnancy, this means that the developing brain can be affected.

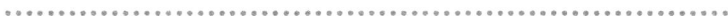

The concentration of alcohol in the mother's blood allows it to be redistributed throughout her body, including storage in various tissues, before it can cause damage. However, this redistribution also means that alcohol can reach the developing brain of her fetus, disrupting normal brain development and leading to the impairments associated with fetal alcohol syndrome.

The first missed period typically occurs about two weeks after conception, which is around the time when the woman may not yet be aware of her pregnancy. If she continues to consume alcohol during this time and only discovers her pregnancy after the second missed period, usually around six weeks after conception, there'd have been three weeks of alcohol exposure for the developing fetus.

They say to be close to your kids and do everything with them to facilitate bonding, but drinking is certainly not one of the things you should be doing with your unborn. Alcohol will impair proper brain development, and the baby will most likely suffer intellectual impairment. Intellectual impairment is only a symptom, and the disease is called fetal alcohol syndrome.

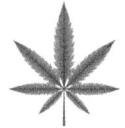

The Link Between Cannabis and the Fetus

Cannabis, like alcohol, can cross the placenta and enter the fetus's bloodstream. This happens because cannabis is a fat-soluble drug, and the placenta is a fatty tissue, so cannabis can dissolve into and through the placenta. It's essential to clarify that the effects of cannabis use during pregnancy on the developing fetus are still an area of ongoing research and debate. While cannabis is known to impact brain development in young adults, its specific effects on the developing brain of a fetus are not yet fully understood. However, we can use our understanding of the human body and other comparable drugs to predict the effects of cannabis on the unborn.

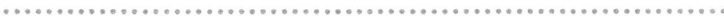

We know that cannabis impairs the full development of the brain, as seen in the "arrested development" of the brains of young adults. We also know cannabis can dissolve in tissues like the brain, bone marrow, and muscle. This means that cannabis can pass from the mother to the unborn via the same mechanism used by alcohol to cause fetal alcohol syndrome.

Some studies have suggested that prenatal exposure to cannabis may be associated with certain risks, including lower birth weight, preterm birth, and potential effects on cognitive and behavioural development. However, it's essential to note that research in this area is complex, and other factors such as co-occurring substance use, health status, lifestyle, and socioeconomic factors may also contribute to these outcomes. Due to the limited and conflicting evidence available, healthcare professionals generally advise pregnant women to avoid cannabis use.

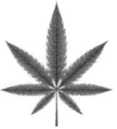

94

Alcohol does significant, irreparable damage to the brain until the blood-brain barrier is fully formed—the eighth week of pregnancy—but cannabis can keep doing damage until the entire brain is fully developed at around twenty-five years of age. It should also be noted that alcohol can still damage brain cells after the eighth week. However, the damage would be less, but it could still be significant if there's chronic alcohol exposure.

Suppose:

1. Alcohol doesn't do much long-term damage to young adults
2. Cannabis impairs brain development in these minors
3. Women who consume alcohol while pregnant put their unborn at an exceptionally high risk of developing fetal alcohol syndrome.
   What do you think would be the effect of cannabis consumption during pregnancy on an unborn child?

Over the last few decades, we've learned that **immunizations** don't cause **autism**. Instead, something else causes the brains of these unborn children to stop growing at some point during **fetal life**. This was discovered when the brains of deceased infants and toddlers with autism were examined microscopically. These brains were found to be at about the same level of development as those of the unborn. How can a brain stop developing before a baby is even born when it's supposed to stop at age twenty-five? From our discussion, does it make sense to point to cannabis as a suspect? This brain damage can also be done by any other fat-soluble drug that interferes with brain structure and function and is taken during or before pregnancy. Can cannabis cause autism? Maybe not, but a suspect until we can prove otherwise.

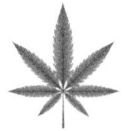

95

HIV and AIDS have been around for over four decades. Little was known about this affliction in
the early eighties. Hundreds, if not thousands,
of people had to die before it was first postulat-
ed that "homosexuals" were the only ones at risk
of this debilitating illness. Several years passed,
and thousands more kicked the bucket before HIV
was considered a threat to anyone receiving blood
from an infected partner or donor.

Even more people faced an early exit to head for
the happy hunting ground before HIV was known
to be a threat to just about anyone who came in
contact with infected blood or body fluids. It took
nearly three decades to develop effective medication for the masses that made infected people less
infectious. HIV was no longer a death sentence it
once was when it first emerged.

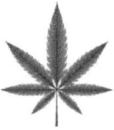

96

If we discover another virus like HIV today, should
we take lessons from the last four decades about
how we dealt with a novel virus and apply them to
fight the new virus, or should we forget everything
and start from scratch? Would we have to start
from the stereotypes of a disease to violent states
of ignorance until we figure it all out? Should our
health care system and authorities just wing it in
the face of new challenges similar to past ones?

People die every day due to a lack of knowledge.
Lack of knowledge can lead some to make poor life
and health decisions, which could end one's life in-
stantly or cause indefinite pain. You don't know
everything, so it's always a good idea to learn to
listen so you can stay out of harm's way. Learn
from the past, make the most of the present, and
leave some hope for the future.

Don't Easily Give Your Heart Away

We now dig deeper into a few concepts that were introduced earlier. This chapter is more technical than the preceding chapters. While this would be a walk in the park for anyone with a good understanding of the basics of medical science, it has been simplified for those with at least a good understanding of high school science. Spending your life without learning how to ride a bicycle may be okay. However, you owe it to yourself to learn things that may harm you or your loved ones, especially those things you can get from your local store.

Understanding Heart Attacks and Strokes

Your brain is a vital organ responsible for controlling and coordinating all functions of your body. It requires a constant supply of oxygen to function correctly. Oxygen is essential for your brain cells (**neurons**) to generate energy and perform their specialized functions. Your brain can't survive for more than four minutes without oxygen. This's why when there's a disruption of blood flow to your brain—a condition known as a **stroke**—every second to help that person becomes critical.

97

When blood flow to your brain is interrupted, your brain cells are deprived of oxygen and nutrients, leading to damage or death. Without timely intervention to restore blood flow, irreversible brain damage can occur.

Recognizing the signs of a stroke and seeking immediate medical attention is crucial. The acronym "FAST" is commonly used to help identify the warning signs of a stroke:

- Face: **Sudden weakness or drooping** on one side of the face.

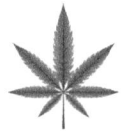

- Arms: **Weakness or numbness** in one arm or leg.
- Speech: Difficulty speaking or understanding speech (**slurred speech**).
- Time: **Time** is of the essence.

If any of these symptoms are observed, it's important to call emergency medical services immediately. Emergency medical professionals can provide appropriate treatment, such as administering clot-dissolving medications or performing procedures to restore blood flow to your brain, depending on the type of stroke.

A heart attack, also known as **myocardial infarction**, occurs when there's a blockage in your **coronary arteries**. Coronary arteries are responsible for supplying oxygen-rich blood to your heart muscle. When a blood clot forms and obstructs blood flow through these arteries, your heart muscle becomes deprived of oxygen.

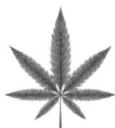

98

Without oxygen, your heart muscle cells start to suffer damage. If blood flow isn't restored promptly, the affected part of your heart muscle can become permanently damaged, leading to complications or even death.

Recognizing the symptoms of a heart attack and taking prompt action is crucial for minimizing damage and improving outcomes. Common symptoms of a heart attack may include:

- **Chest pain or discomfort**: This can manifest as a feeling of pressure, tightness, or squeezing in your chest. It may also radiate to your arms, jaw, neck, back, or stomach.
- **Shortness of breath**: Difficulty breathing or feeling breathless, often accompanying chest discomfort.
- Sweating: **Profuse sweating** unrelated to physical activity or temperature.

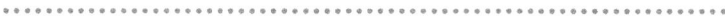

- **Nausea or vomiting**: Some people may experience these symptoms during a heart attack.
- Light-headedness or dizziness: F**eeling faint or lightheaded**.

If you or someone around you experiences symptoms suggestive of a heart attack, it's important to call emergency medical services right away. While waiting for medical assistance to arrive, chewing and swallowing a baby **aspirin** (if not allergic) can help inhibit the formation of more **blood clots**.

Making Red Blood Cells

Red blood cells (RBCs) are recycled every 120 days, so you always make RBCs as they constantly turn over. When making RBCs, you typically start with one cell that divides similarly to **binary fission**; that is, one cell divides into 2, then 2 to 4, 4 to 8, 16, 32, and so on. This division process requires an essential B vitamin called **folate** or B9. Folate can be found in a variety of natural food sources, including:

99

- **Leafy green vegetables**: Vegetables like spinach, broccoli, kale, and lettuce are excellent sources of methyl folate.
- **Citrus fruits**: Fruits like oranges, lemons, grape fruits, and strawberries provide a good amount of folate.
- **Legumes**: Lentils, black beans, chickpeas, and other legumes are rich in folate.
- **Nuts and seeds**: Sunflower seeds, almonds, peanuts, and flaxseeds are examples of nuts and seeds that contain methyl folate.
- **Meat**: Organ meats like liver and kidney are exceptionally high in folate.
- **Eggs**: Eggs are a good source of folate, especially in the yolk.
- **Dairy products**: Milk, cheese, and yogurt can contribute to your folate intake.

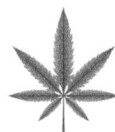

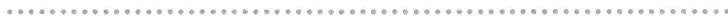

It's important to note that the folate content in food can vary depending on factors such as soil quality and storage conditions. Additionally, cooking methods can affect folate levels, with prolonged cooking or high heat potentially reducing folate content. Therefore, consuming folate-rich foods in their raw or lightly cooked form can help preserve their folate content.

In cell division, your body can't use **methyl folate** in that form because of the "methyl" group attached to it. In that case, you'll need another B vitamin, cobalamin or B12. The purpose of cobalamin in this particular setup is to change methyl folate to folate by taking away the methyl group from methyl folate. When B12 takes this methyl group from methyl folate, it'll then pass it to another substance called **homocysteine**.

Homocysteine is an amino acid, a component of proteins. Elevated levels of homocysteine in your blood, also known as **hyperhomocysteinemia**, are associated with an increased risk of various health conditions such as heart attacks and strokes.

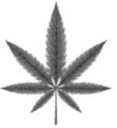

100

Usually, homocysteine is rapidly converted to harmless compounds in your body through a series of reactions that require the presence of vitamins B12, B9, and B6. However, when these vitamins aren't available in sufficient amounts, homocysteine can accumulate in your blood, leading to hyperhomocysteinemia.

Several factors can contribute to elevated homocysteine levels, including:

- **Genetics**: Some individuals may have **genetic mutations** that affect the enzymes responsible for homocysteine metabolism, leading to increased levels.
- **Nutritional deficiencies**: Inadequate intake or absorption of vitamins B12, B9, and B6 can impair the proper metabolism of homocysteine. These vitamins play a crucial

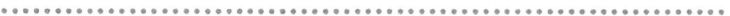

role in converting homocysteine to other compounds.
- **Smoking**: Smoking has been found to increase homocysteine levels in the blood.
- **Alcohol consumption**: Excessive alcohol consumption can interfere with the metabolism of vitamins involved in homocysteine processing.
- **Age**: Homocysteine levels tend to increase with age, possibly due to nutrient absorption and metabolism changes.

When vitamin B12 gives homocysteine the methyl group it took from B9, homocysteine will be converted to a harmless substance called **methionine**. Methionine will go on to make proteins that are vital for your body. In the end, you'll have free folate that'll go on to aid in cell division, methionine that will make proteins, and free cobalamin that will go back to process another methyl folate or return to participate in other **biochemical reactions**.

Note that at the end of this process, all substances are converted to what your body can use without causing harm or initiating chaos in your blood. It's also pertinent to note that B12 isn't used up in the process. B12 can be reused repeatedly and won't be depleted by this process. From this, you can see how a vitamin B9 or B12 deficiency can lead to lethal problems. Without methyl folate or cobalamine, homocysteine can't be processed and thus accumulates in your body, resulting in heart attacks or strokes.

The Relationship Between Hypoxia and Hemoglobin Levels

In the chapter **"Firing up the Bag of Wind"** we explored how changes in gases in your lungs can lead to a condition called **hypoxia**, where there's a reduced level of oxygen available. Since your body relies on oxygen for proper functioning, it has a clever mecha-

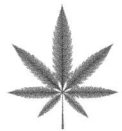

nism to counter this challenge: increasing the production of RBCs.

When there's a decrease in oxygen reaching your cells due to changes in lung gases, your body responds by boosting the production of RBCs. The rationale behind this response is simple: if the usual amount of RBCs isn't delivering enough oxygen to your cells, why not produce more RBCs to ensure an adequate oxygen supply? This's similar to stocking up on food supplies when there's a possibility of food shortages.

In Medicine, it's well-recognized that hypoxia can stimulate the production of **hemoglobin**. Hemoglobin is the component of RBCs responsible for carrying oxygen to your tissues. When your body senses hypoxia, it initiates mechanisms to increase the production of RBCs, leading to higher hemoglobin levels.

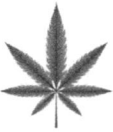

102

Under normal circumstances, the hemoglobin concentration in adult males typically ranges from 15 to 17 grams per deciliter (g/dL). However, hemoglobin levels can rise even higher in individuals who experience prolonged periods of hypoxia, such as those living at high altitudes or individuals with certain medical conditions. In cases of **chronic hypoxia**, normal hemoglobin levels as high as 21 g/dL have been observed.

It's worth noting that there can be differences in hemoglobin levels between males and females. On average, females tend to have hemoglobin levels at least 2 g/dL lower than their male counterparts. Various factors, including hormonal, physical, and genetic factors, influence these differences.

Here're some factors that contribute to the observed differences in hemoglobin levels between men and women:

- **RBC count**: Men generally have a higher RBC count compared to women. This's partly attributed to hormonal differences and the effects of testosterone, which stimulates RBC production. The higher RBC count in men contributes to their overall higher hemoglobin levels.
- **Muscle mass and oxygen demand**: Men tend to have more muscle mass than women, and muscles require a greater supply of oxygen to function optimally. To meet the increased oxygen demand, your body produces more RBCs and increases hemoglobin levels to enhance oxygen-carrying capacity.
- **Blood volume**: Men typically have a larger blood volume than women. With a larger blood volume, more RBCs and hemoglobin circulate in your bloodstream, which can lead to higher hemoglobin levels.
- **Menstrual blood loss**: Women experience menstrual bleeding, which leads to monthly blood loss. This blood loss can result in decreased RBCs and hemoglobin levels, potentially contributing to lower hemoglobin levels in women compared to men. Menstrual blood loss can also increase some women's risk of developing anemia.

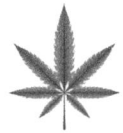

103

It's important to note that these factors contribute to the observed differences in hemoglobin levels between men and women at a population level. However, there's variability within each gender, and individual variations can exist. Other factors such as age, health conditions, and lifestyle can also influence hemoglobin levels.

Certain conditions and diseases can affect hemoglobin levels, either increasing or decreasing them. For

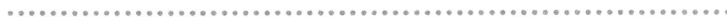

example, chronic lung diseases, such as COPD, can cause low oxygen levels in your blood, leading to increased production of RBCs and higher hemoglobin levels as a compensatory response. On the other hand, certain types of anemia can result in low hemoglobin levels due to decreased RBC production or increased RBC destruction.

Marathon runners, who engage in prolonged intense exercise, can experience temporary hypoxia due to the increased oxygen demands during exercise. People who reside at high altitudes, where the oxygen concentration in the air is lower, may also develop chronic hypoxia over time. Additionally, smoking can lead to chronic hypoxia as tobacco smoke contains carbon monoxide, which reduces the **oxygen-carrying capacity** of hemoglobin.

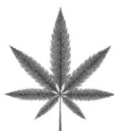

It's important to emphasize that high hemoglobin levels alone don't necessarily indicate a health problem. However, a healthcare professional should evaluate persistently elevated or decreased levels to determine the underlying cause and ensure appropriate management.

104

Smoking, folate, and hemoglobin

If smoking can cause hypoxia, and hypoxia can lead to an increase in the production of RBCs, the increased cell division required to produce more RBCs can easily lead to a depletion of your folate. The problem isn't only the resulting folate deficiency but the effect that a folate deficiency can have on subsequent reactions. Without folate to bring the methyl group in the process described in the section **"Making Red Blood Cells"** cobalamin is left sitting idle, waiting to carry a methyl group that may or may not show up. Further down the chain, homocysteine is pissed off because it won't get its methyl group from cobalamin to form a non-toxic chemical, methionine.

The end result of all this is an increase in homocysteine levels in your blood, and this homocysteine will promote the clumping of RBCs, causing clots within blood vessels. As with the rest of your blood, these clots will be pumped throughout your blood vessels. However, due to their size, blood clots will eventually get into tiny blood vessels, where they'll cause a blockage. If this blockage happens in a blood vessel in your brain, we call that a stroke—and if it occurs in a blood vessel that feeds your heart muscle, we call that a heart attack. Strokes and heart attacks have several other causes beyond this book's scope. However, please note that this chain of events that leads to a heart attack or stroke started with smoke inhalation, which caused a notable decrease in your blood oxygen concentration.

Some people may think getting folate supplements is a brilliant idea to counteract their smoking habits, but there are two main problems with that.

- **Folate supplements and cobalamin interaction**: It's important to note that folate supplements alone may not address the underlying issue of elevated homocysteine levels in individuals who smoke. Cobalamin is required to convert homocysteine into methionine, a non-toxic substance. The detoxification process is impaired without sufficient cobalamin, leading to increased homocysteine levels. Therefore, simply supplementing with folate may help with cell division to produce more RBCs but may not be adequate to lower homocysteine levels if cobalamin is deficient. Additionally, some folate supplements sold don't contain the methyl group cobalamin needs to give to homocysteine to detoxify it into methionine.

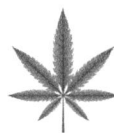

105

- **Folate and cancer risk**: While folate is essential for cell division and growth, it's crucial to approach folate supplementation cautiously in individuals at high risk of developing cancer, such as smokers. Some studies suggest that high levels of folate intake, particularly from supplements, may potentially promote the growth of existing cancer cells.

While research specifically focusing on cannabis smoking and cardiovascular health is limited compared to studies on tobacco smoking, there's evidence to suggest potential risks.

The combustion of tobacco or cannabis can lead to inhaling harmful substances and reducing oxygen supply, contributing to hypoxia and subsequent cardiovascular complications. It's worth noting that cannabis smoke contains many of the same toxic compounds and carcinogens as tobacco smoke, albeit in different proportions.

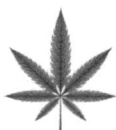

106

It's essential to acknowledge that individual responses to cannabis smoking can vary. The overall impact on cardiovascular health may be influenced by factors such as frequency of use, dose, duration, underlying health conditions, and co-use with other substances.

Two guys were sitting on a park bench. They looked around and found no one but birds and trees, so they decided to fire one up. These guys were somewhat nervous about the whole thing because they were trying weed for the first time.

Twenty minutes later, they were still sitting on the bench, but in a different universe. This was the best and the freakiest of times. They were both feeling something but unsure how to ask the other friend if they felt the same. In the end, one of them asked, "When did it get so dark all of a sudden?" The other friend freaked out even more and exclaimed, "It's still the middle of daylight!" This sparked a massive argument between the two that went on for several minutes.

In the middle of all this, they found a potential solution. They saw someone walking towards them. They didn't know or care if this person would've been a police officer. All they wanted was for their issue to be resolved. This guy walking towards them turned out to be an ordinary citizen but might've been floating higher than they were. When they explained their story and the dilemma, they asked the guy, "Can you please tell us if this is day or night?" Without hesitation, the guy replied, "I'm sorry, guys, but I don't live around here."

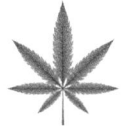

107

I Might Be Crazy, But I'm Loving It!

Breaking Down Depression

Depression, the uninvited guest in your mind, is no laughing matter. Let's shed some light on this weighty topic with valuable information. Depression is like a rain cloud that hangs over a person, dampening their spirits and making life feel like a never-ending gloomy day.

Imagine feeling persistently sad, empty, or hopeless, as if the sun has disappeared from the sky. Activities that once brought joy and excitement now seem as appealing as a soggy sandwich. Sleep becomes a fickle friend, either playing hard to get or overstaying its welcome like an unwelcome houseguest. Concentration and decision-making become as challenging as solving a Rubik's Cube blindfolded.

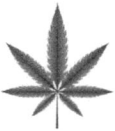

Feelings of worthlessness and guilt can weigh as heavy as a bag of rocks. At the same time, your appetite goes on a rollercoaster ride, either vanishing completely or tempting you to indulge in all the snacks your heart desires. Fatigue becomes your constant companion, draining your energy faster than a phone battery on a YouTube binge. And if that's not enough, thoughts of death or suicide may cloud your mind, turning even the simplest moments into a dark labyrinth.

Brain chemicals like serotonin and dopamine play a significant role in **mood regulation**. When they misbehave, they can contribute to the blues. Life events, both big and small, can act as triggers, like stumbling upon a banana peel in the journey of life. Medical conditions can also team up with depression, forming an unholy alliance that makes everything feel twice as heavy.

Depression can be caused by a combination of genetic,

biological, environmental, and psychological factors. It can be triggered by a traumatic event or life change, such as losing a loved one, a relationship break-up, a job loss, or stagnation in love, life, or work. It can also be associated with certain medical conditions such as chronic pain, heart disease, or stroke. In some cases, the cause of depression is not clear.

But fear not, my friends! Just as laughter is the best medicine for the soul, there's hope and help for those grappling with depression. Seeking the guidance of mental health professionals is like having a trusty sidekick to navigate the stormy seas of emotions. They can offer therapy, a safe space to explore thoughts and feelings, and provide coping strategies to weather the storm.

Sometimes, medication swoops in as a superhero, restoring the delicate balance of brain chemicals. And don't underestimate the power of lifestyle changes! Engaging in activities that bring joy, exercising those happy **endorphins**, and surrounding yourself with a supportive social network can be as uplifting as finding a 50-dollar bill in your pocket while doing laundry.

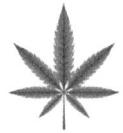

109

The Highs and Lows of Effective Depression Treatments

Cannabis is known to give a sense of physical and psychological relief, which is known as "being high." This **euphoric effect** of cannabis remains one of the most sought-after effects of the drug. Now, imagine a world where we could isolate only the euphoric effect of cannabis and inject it into every food item. We'd have a planet full of overweight, blissed-out individuals floating around with permanent smiles and a relentless craving for snacks.

If cannabis can provide that sought-after euphoria, it stands to reason that it may benefit those feeling physically or psychologically tense. It's like finding a hidden oasis in the desert of stress and worries. In fact, other drugs used to treat depression and anxiety work by similar principles.

Let's be clear, though. No drug, not even cannabis, can magically cure the heartache of losing a loved one, the sting of a relationship break-up, the blow of a job loss, or the feeling of being stuck in life's monotony. However, **antidepressants** and other **mood-altering medications** can work their magic by tinkering with the delicate chemistry of your brain. They offer a temporary respite, like a much-needed vacation from your troubles. They can bring a sense of peace or pleasure that helps you momentarily forget about your problems and find solace in the depths of your mind.

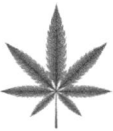

Imagine this scenario: the drug wears off, and those pesky problems—the ones that seem to have a knack for sticking around—reappear with unwavering persistence. And what's the next step? You guessed it, reaching for another pill in pursuit of another fleeting moment of respite. It's a never-ending cycle of pill-popping behaviour that can become addictive like a hamster endlessly running on its wheel without ever reaching a destination. It's like expecting the soothing properties of a band-aid to magically heal a broken bone.

110

The underlying assumption or hope is that these pills will enable you to better cope with life's challenges. We all yearn for the ability to navigate the stormy seas of loss, heartbreak, and stagnation with greater ease and resilience. However, the reality is that relying solely on medication to address these deep-seated issues may not be the silver bullet you hope for.

Consider the countless individuals who have been on these "happy pills" for years, if not decades. Their stories serve as a sobering reminder that something may be amiss with the pill-popping approach to treating depression. It's a delicate dance between seeking relief and unintentionally falling into a cycle of dependency on medication.

It's pertinent to acknowledge that the journey to addressing mental health concerns requires a comprehensive approach that extends beyond simply popping a pill. While medication can be valuable in managing symptoms, combining it with other therapeutic interventions is crucial. This might include counselling, therapy, lifestyle modifications, and cultivating a robust support network. By addressing the underlying issues and developing healthy coping mechanisms, you can begin to pave a path toward long-lasting healing.

Basic Principles of Psychoanalysis From a Cannabis Perspective

Aside from its therapeutic use, which can potentially help millions of people, cannabis is mainly taken just for fun, with no therapeutic purpose. During intoxication, various physiological and cognitive functions are affected, including perception, coordination, and cognitive processing. These altered states of consciousness can give individuals a sense of euphoria, relaxation, and varied sensory experiences.

111

One of the notable effects of cannabis intoxication is a general slowing down of body functions. People may feel a sense of physical and mental relaxation, which can lead to a sedative-like state. This can manifest as individuals sitting or lying down, sometimes experiencing a distorted perception of time and space. Metaphorically speaking, they may feel like they are floating on "cloud nine," hence the colloquial phrase "being high." Additionally, **impaired coordination** and cognitive functions can pose safety risks, particularly when engaging in activities such as driving or swimming.

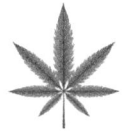

The extremes of this behaviour in people in this state are what is of concern as they can range from breaking relationships to breaking the law. To understand this, we need to go and look at part of Sigmund Freud's theory of **psychoanalysis**, an idea in psychology and a method of psychotherapy. Don't worry; we'll only look at what will help us understand the psychological implications of cannabis, the thought processes when someone is "high." While we'll only touch upon the basics, it can help illuminate the interplay between free thinking and social limitations.

According to Freud's theory of psychoanalysis, individuals' thoughts and behaviours are influenced by both their inner desires and societal expectations. A compromise exists between freely expressing one's thoughts and conforming to social norms, commonly observed as "normal behaviour" within a given society. Psychoanalysis posits that mental disorders arise from unconscious conflicts within an individual's psyche. These conflicts can be brought to conscious awareness and resolved through techniques such as free association and interpretation.

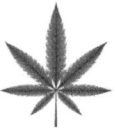

When someone is under the influence of cannabis, their thought processes may become altered. The drug's psychoactive properties can impact perception, cognition, and emotional experiences. These altered mental states may temporarily loosen the constraints imposed by societal expectations, allowing for more uninhibited thoughts and behaviours. Cannabis intoxication can lead to a sense of increased introspection, creativity, and **divergent thinking**.

However, it's important to note that while cannabis may temporarily alter thought processes, it doesn't necessarily address underlying unconscious conflicts or psychological issues. The effects of cannabis intoxication are temporary and may not provide a long-term resolution for mental disorders or emotional challenges. It's crucial to approach the use of cannabis, whether recreationally or therapeutically, with an understanding of its limitations and potential risks.

In psychoanalysis, the concept of the **psyche** is divided into three parts: the **id**, the **superego**, and the **ego**. Each part plays a distinct role in shaping your thoughts, behaviours, and decision-making processes.
The id is the primitive and instinctual part of the psyche. It operates on the pleasure principle, seeking immediate gratification of your desires and needs. The id is unconscious and not influenced by reality or the consequences of your actions. It represents our basic drives and urges.

On the other hand, the superego is the **moral** and **ethical** part of the psyche. It develops during childhood and is shaped by your experiences and the values you learn from your parents, society, and culture. The superego acts as your conscience and guides you in distinguishing between right and wrong. It represents your internalized societal and moral standards.

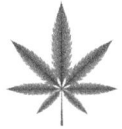

113

The ego serves as the rational and realistic part of the psyche. It operates on the reality principle and mediates between the demands of the id and the demands of the external world. The ego enables us to think, reason, and make decisions. Its role is to balance the conflicting demands of the id and superego, taking into account the laws of society and the constraints of reality.

According to psychoanalysis, these three parts of the psyche are in constant interaction and often in conflict with each other. The ego's task is to manage and navigate these conflicts, finding compromises that satisfy both the demands of the id and the superego. When the ego successfully balances these competing forces, it allows for adaptive and socially acceptable behaviour.

To paint a picture: a man sees an attractive woman and desperately wants to lay his hands on her right away. The man's immediate desire to physically engage with the woman represents the id's impulsive and pleasure-seeking nature. However, his understanding of societal norms, legal boundaries, and respect for the woman's autonomy represents the influence of the superego.

The ego comes into play to find a balance between these conflicting forces. The ego considers the reality of the situation, including social norms and legal constraints. It seeks a compromise that allows for a socially acceptable action. In this case, the ego may guide the man to respectfully approach the woman, ask her out, or politely compliment her.

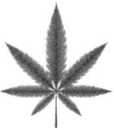

114

It's important to note that the outcomes can vary depending on the individual and their unique psychological makeup. Sometimes the id's desires may prevail, leading to impulsive and inappropriate actions. Other times, the superego's strict adherence to societal rules may prevent any action at all. However, in many cases, the ego strives to find a balance between these extremes, resulting in socially acceptable behaviour that respects the individual's desires and society's values.

When under the influence of cannabis, the inhibitory functions of the superego can be suppressed, leading to a decreased ability to regulate and control your impulses. This can result in behaviours that are more aligned with the id's immediate desires and less influenced by societal norms or consequences. Remember the guy we met earlier? Suppose that guy is "high" on cannabis, and his superego is inhibited. In that case, you can imagine a guy being whacked by a purse and flying into the bushes because he followed his id without the guidance of the superego.

This's essentially the same phenomenon observed with alcohol Intoxication. Since these drugs are supposed to slow you down but somehow allow you to act wild, this phenomenon is called **paradoxical disinhibition**. It refers to the apparent contradiction of experiencing a state of relaxation or sedation while at the same time displaying uninhibited or wild behaviour.

Understanding Your Brain, and Your Brain on Cannabis

While the so-called "good" effects of cannabis on relieving anxiety are all sought after, this drug tends to come with some undesirable adverse effects on your mind. Your brain essentially has three components:

- The physical structure is known as **neurons**.
- The wiring that connects the neurons is called **neurotransmitters**.
- The functionality that comes as a result of those connections.

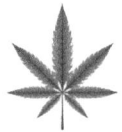

115

Neurotransmitters are chemical messengers that transmit signals between neurons in your brain. They're crucial in various cognitive and behavioural processes, including mood regulation, memory, and cognition. We don't feel the neurons or the neurotransmitters, but the functionality is what we experience because of these connections; feelings, thoughts, memory, comprehension, etc.

Without neurons or the proper arrangement of these neurons, you may not have the appropriate neurotransmitters, which can result in impaired brain function. The endocannabinoid system (ECS) is involved in regulating neurotransmitter release and

synaptic function. Once it stimulates the ECS, THC can affect the balance and functioning of neurotransmitters in your brain, particularly dopamine, serotonin, and **gamma-aminobutyric** acid (GABA). These neurotransmitters affect mood regulation, reward processing, anxiety, and other cognitive functions.

Excessive or chronic cannabis use has been associated with potential disruptions in the normal functioning of neurotransmitters. For example, it has been suggested that long-term cannabis use may decrease dopamine levels in certain brain regions, which can contribute to changes in motivation and reward sensitivity.

Additionally, cannabis use has been linked to alterations in serotonin levels, which may impact mood regulation and potentially affect anxiety and depression. With billions of neurons and over half a dozen neurotransmitters that need to be replenished in appropriate amounts at appropriate times in your brain, a lot can impact the proper functioning of your brain.

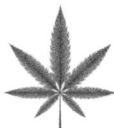

116

Neuropsychiatry is a branch of medicine that combines the fields of neurology and psychiatry, aiming to understand the relationship between brain structure, function, and mental disorders. Your brain is an incredibly complex organ composed of billions of neurons that communicate with each other through intricate networks.

Proper brain function relies on the precise balance and regulation of neurotransmitters. Different neurotransmitters have specific roles in modulating various cognitive, emotional, and behavioural processes. For example, serotonin is involved in mood regulation, dopamine is associated with reward and motivation, and GABA helps regulate inhibitory processes in the brain.

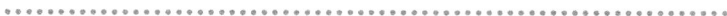

When there're imbalances or disruptions in the functioning of neurons or neurotransmitters, it can impact brain function and potentially contribute to the development of mental disorders. Conditions such as depression, anxiety disorders, **schizophrenia**, and others have been linked to abnormalities in neuronal circuits and neurotransmitter systems.

The study of psychology, on the other hand, focuses on understanding human behaviour, cognition, and the processes underlying thoughts and emotions. While neuropsychiatry examines the biological basis of mental disorders, psychology delves into the psychological, social, and environmental factors that influence behaviour and cognitive processes. Both fields, neuropsychiatry and psychology, contribute valuable insights into understanding the complexities of your brain and mind, aiming to improve mental health and well-being.

Substance Use and Abuse, and Disease and Disorders

117

Your brain is a sensitive organ easily susceptible to damage or impairment, and the resulting effects can vary from benign to debilitating. Over time, there've been links between certain drugs and neurotransmitters, and certain diseases. For example,

- **Serotonin deficiency**: Serotonin is a neurotransmitter that regulates mood, anxiety, and sleep. A serotonin deficiency can lead to depression, anxiety disorders, and **insomnia**.
- **Dopamine deficiency**: Dopamine is a neurotransmitter that regulates movement, motivation, and reward. A dopamine deficiency can lead to **Parkinson's disease**, schizophrenia, and **attention deficit hyperactivity disorder** (ADHD).
- **Acetylcholine deficiency**: Acetylcholine

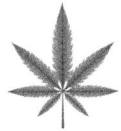

is a neurotransmitter that plays a role in regulating memory and learning. An acetylcholine deficiency can lead to conditions such as **Alzheimer's** disease and other forms of **dementia**.

- **GABA deficiency**: GABA is a neurotransmitter that plays a role in regulating anxiety and stress. A deficiency in GABA can lead to conditions such as anxiety disorders, insomnia, and **seizures**.
- **Norepinephrine deficiency**: **Norepinephrine** is a neurotransmitter that regulates arousal, attention, and mood. A deficiency in norepinephrine can lead to conditions such as depression and **attention deficit disorder** (ADD).
- **Cannabis**: Long-term use of marijuana can lead to addiction, and can cause mental health conditions such as anxiety, depression, and psychosis. It also can lead to respiratory problems and lung infections from smoking.
- **Cocaine**: Long-term use of cocaine can lead to addiction, and can cause mental health conditions such as anxiety, depression, and paranoia. It also can cause heart attacks, strokes, and seizures. Cocaine has been linked to Parkinson's disease.
- **Opioids**: Long-term use of opioids can lead to addiction, and can cause mental health conditions such as anxiety, depression, and psychosis. It also can cause respiratory problems and overdose.
- **Amphetamines**: Long-term use of amphetamines can lead to addiction, and can cause mental health conditions such as anxiety, depression, and psychosis. It also can cause heart attacks, strokes, and seizures.
- **Alcohol**: Long-term use of alcohol can lead to addiction, and can cause mental health conditions such as anxiety, depression, and psychosis. It also can cause liver disease, **pancreatitis** and cancer.

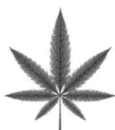

While most individuals who use cannabis won't develop psychosis, research has shown an increased risk, especially for those who use cannabis frequently and at high doses. Studies have found that cannabis use, particularly in individuals predisposed or with a personal or family history of mental health disorders, can contribute to developing or exacerbating psychotic symptoms. The risk is higher for individuals who start using cannabis at a young age, as the adolescent brain is still undergoing critical developmental processes.

The exact mechanisms by which cannabis use may trigger or worsen psychosis aren't fully understood, but they're thought to involve the interaction between cannabinoids and the brain's neurotransmitter systems, including dopamine. Cannabis use has been shown to increase dopamine release in certain brain regions, disrupting the delicate balance of neurotransmitters and potentially contributing to psychosis.

Understanding Psychosis

Psychosis is a complex symptom associated with various mental health conditions and other factors. It's characterized by losing contact with reality and can significantly impact your thoughts, perceptions, and behaviour. Prompt diagnosis and appropriate treatment are crucial for managing and addressing psychosis effectively.

Individuals experiencing psychosis may have difficulty distinguishing between reality and fiction, and may experience **hallucinations** and **delusions**. Hallucinations are perceptions that aren't based on reality. They can include hearing voices, seeing things, or experiencing other sensory distortions. Delusions are fixed false beliefs that an individual holds despite evidence to the contrary. These can include beliefs that one is being persecuted, has special powers or abilities, or is in control of events that are not actually in their control.

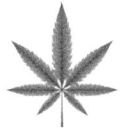

119

Psychosis can be a symptom of several mental health conditions, including schizophrenia, **bipolar disorder**, and severe depression. Substance abuse, medical conditions, or brain injuries can also cause it. Its onset can be sudden or gradual, and symptoms can range from mild to severe. Treatment for psychosis typically involves a combination of medication and psychotherapy. **Antipsychotic medication** can help reduce the symptoms of psychosis, while **psychotherapy** can help the individual better understand and cope with reality.

Substance-induced psychosis, which can occur as a result of drug use, including cannabis use, requires addressing both the substance abuse issue and the associated psychotic symptoms. Treatment may involve:

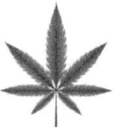

- Substance abuse treatment programs.
- Detoxification if necessary.
- Therapy aimed at managing both the substance use disorder and psychosis.

120

It's important to note that psychosis is a serious condition, and individuals experiencing psychosis should seek professional help as soon as possible. Early intervention and treatment can improve the outcome, help the individual regain contact with reality, and improve their quality of life.

Cannabis-induced Psychosis

"What happened to that kid from next door since he started smoking weed? He's become so weird that he freaks me out," said a curious neighbour. How exactly do these teens go from being high to being crazy? Is there really a link between cannabis and psychosis, or is it a small fluke blown out of proportion? Do we have a real threat here, or are more people just trying to get in the way of good people trying to have a good time?

The basis of the link between cannabis and psychosis goes back a few discussions. Cannabis is a fat-soluble drug, which means when smoked, eaten, or put under your tongue, it'll first go into your blood before it distributes to fatty tissues like your brain, muscle, and bone marrow. The tissue of interest here is your brain.

When cannabis is consumed, the active compounds in the plant, such as THC, enter your bloodstream and are distributed throughout your body, including your brain. THC is a fat-soluble molecule, which means it can easily cross the blood-brain barrier and enter your brain tissue.

Once in your brain, THC interacts with the endocannabinoid system. The endocannabinoid system impacts the balance of neurotransmitters in your brain, including dopamine, serotonin, and **glutamate**, which are neurotransmitters implicated in mental health conditions.

The effects of THC on your brain can be both pleasurable and potentially disruptive. The pleasant effects are often associated with the euphoric or "high" feeling people experience when using cannabis. However, the disruptive effects can include memory, attention, and cognitive function impairments, which may be more pronounced in heavy or frequent cannabis users.

It's believed that THC's interaction with the endocannabinoid system, specifically the CB1 receptors in your brain, may contribute to developing or exacerbating psychotic symptoms in vulnerable individuals. Various factors, including genetic predisposition, family history of psychosis, early age of cannabis use, and frequency and potency of cannabis use, can influence this vulnerability.

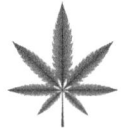

What is myelin?

The **myelin sheath** is a fatty protective coating that surrounds and insulates nerve fibres, including those in your brain. It primarily comprises lipids, precisely a type of lipid called myelin lipids. The myelin sheath is essential for the proper functioning of your nervous system.

The primary function of the myelin sheath is to increase the speed and efficiency of **nerve impulse transmission**. When an electrical signal, called an **action potential**, is generated in a neuron, it travels down the nerve fibre. The myelin sheath acts as an **insulator**, preventing the electrical signal from leaking out and ensuring that it efficiently propagates along the nerve fibre.

In addition to enhancing nerve impulse conduction, the myelin sheath provides nerve fibres protection and support. It helps to maintain the structural integrity of neurons and prevents damage or injury to the delicate nerve fibres.

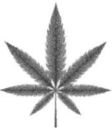

122

Disruptions or damage to the myelin sheath can significantly affect brain function and overall nervous system functioning. Conditions that involve the loss or damage of the myelin sheath, such as **multiple sclerosis**, can lead to impaired nerve impulse transmission and various neurological symptoms.

Multiple sclerosis (MS) is an **autoimmune disorder** in which your immune system mistakenly attacks the myelin sheath in the **central nervous system** (brain and spinal cord). This immune response leads to inflammation and damage to the myelin, disrupting the normal functioning of the nerves.

As a result of the damaged myelin sheath, the transmission of nerve impulses is impaired, leading to a wide range of symptoms depending on the location and extent of the damage. Common symptoms of MS include muscle weakness, numbness or tingling sensations, problems with coordination and balance, fatigue, difficulties with vision, and cognitive changes.

The exact cause of MS is still not fully understood. However, it's believed to involve a combination of genetic and environmental factors. While your immune system's role in attacking the myelin sheath is well-established, the triggers for this autoimmune response are complex and may involve interactions with various environmental factors.

The **myelination** process, which is the formation of the myelin sheath around nerve fibres, is influenced by several environmental factors. Adequate levels of certain nutrients, such as **essential fatty acids** and **vitamins**, are necessary to synthesize and maintain myelin. Regular physical activity has also been shown to promote myelin production and support overall brain health. On the other hand, chronic stress and certain lifestyle factors, such as poor diet and sedentary behaviour, may negatively impact myelin health.

Maintaining a healthy lifestyle that includes a balanced diet, regular exercise, stress management, and avoiding harmful substances is vital for supporting the integrity of the myelin sheath and promoting overall cognitive and physical well-being.

123

Myelin and the Developing Human

The myelination process starts during fetal development and continues through childhood and adolescence. Cannabis is easily stored in myelin, among other places in your brain. Can you spot the possible link between cannabis and harm to an unborn child, infants, toddlers, and teenagers here?

The potential effects of cannabis on the developing brain, particularly in unborn children, infants, toddlers, and teenagers, is an area of active research and scientific debate. While it's critical to approach this

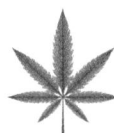

topic with caution due to the complexity of brain development and the many factors that can influence it, evidence suggests that exposure to cannabis during these critical stages of development may have adverse effects.

The developing brain undergoes rapid changes and is particularly sensitive to external influences. The endocannabinoid system, which is involved in various physiological processes, including brain development and function, is also susceptible to the effects of cannabis. THC can cross the placental barrier and reach the developing fetus, potentially impacting its growth.

Studies have suggested that **prenatal** exposure to cannabis may be associated with an increased risk of certain developmental and behavioural issues in children, such as impaired cognitive function, attention and behavioural problems, and an increased likelihood of developing psychiatric disorders later in life. However, it's essential to note that the research in this area is complex.

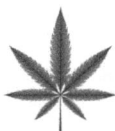

124

Why Cannabis Exposure to Minors Should Be a Big Deal?

In infants, toddlers, and teenagers, the impact of cannabis can also be significant. During these stages, the developing brain continues to undergo crucial processes, including myelination. Disrupting these processes through exposure to cannabis, especially high THC concentrations, may interfere with normal brain development and have long-term consequences.

It's worth emphasizing that the developing brain is vulnerable and that introducing foreign substances like cannabis during critical periods of growth and myelination raises concerns. If you have a drug (foreign to your body) come in to live right next to one of the most sensitive cells in your body, what do you think will happen? What are the chances this particular chemical won't cause any trouble for the neurons if it stays there? Think of this as a drug lord known for pushing drugs to minors who is now moving in next to an elementary school. Cannabis is the drug lord, and the elementary school is the neuron in a fetus, infant, toddler, or teenager.

The Link Between Cannabis and Schizophrenia

The relationship between cannabis use and schizophrenia is a complex and debated topic in psychiatry. While research has shown a consistent association between cannabis use and an increased risk of developing schizophrenia or psychotic symptoms, establishing a causal link has been challenging.

It's important to note that schizophrenia is a multifactorial disorder influenced by a combination of genetic, environmental, and neurobiological factors. Cannabis use is considered an environmental factor that may contribute to developing or exacerbating schizophrenia in vulnerable individuals.

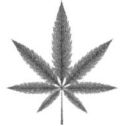

125

Several hypotheses have been proposed to explain the potential link between cannabis and schizophrenia. One theory suggests that cannabis use, particularly during adolescence when the brain is still developing, may interact with genetic factors and disrupt your brain's normal development and functioning, including the dopamine system. Dopamine dysregulation is thought to play a role in the **pathophysiology** of schizophrenia.

Cannabis use has been found to increase the release of dopamine in certain brain regions, which could potentially contribute to the onset of psychotic symptoms. Additionally, the high concentration of THC is believed to play a role in triggering or exacerbating psychosis in susceptible individuals.

While these hypotheses provide a plausible explanation for the association between cannabis use and schizophrenia, it's also essential to consider other factors. Factors such as genetic vulnerability, early-life stress, other substance use, and social factors can also contribute to the development of schizophrenia and interact with cannabis use.

It's worth noting that not everyone who uses cannabis will develop schizophrenia, and individuals with schizophrenia may not necessarily have a history of cannabis use.

What is Schizophrenia?

Schizophrenia is a chronic and serious mental disorder characterized by a disconnection from reality. The name literally translates to a "split personality." Think of this split personality as having one leg in reality and the other leg in your own world. Schizophrenia affects how a person thinks, feels, and behaves. Symptoms can be categorized into two types: positive symptoms and negative symptoms.

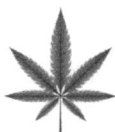

126

Positive symptoms refer to the presence of abnormal experiences and behaviours. Think of these symptoms as adding to someone's personality. Things you DO now but didn't do before, such as:

- **Hallucinations**: hearing, seeing, feeling, or smelling things that aren't there
- **Delusions**: false beliefs that are not based on reality
- **Disordered thinking**: trouble organizing thoughts, connecting them or making sense of them
- **Agitation or catatonia**: abnormal movements or lack of movements

Negative symptoms refer to the absence of normal experiences and behaviours. Think of these symptoms as things you used to do or things normal for most people, but you DON'T do anymore, such as:

- Lack of motivation
- Lack of emotional expression
- Lack of interest in social activities
- Difficulty in initiating and sustaining goal-directed behaviour

It's important to note that symptoms of schizophrenia can vary among individuals, and not all individuals with schizophrenia will experience the same symptoms. The severity and combination of symptoms can also differ over time.

Treatment for schizophrenia often involves a combination of antipsychotic medication, psychosocial interventions, and support services. Early intervention and ongoing management can help individuals with schizophrenia manage their symptoms, improve their overall functioning, and enhance their quality of life.

127

Schizophrenia typically develops in the late teenage years or early adulthood. The onset of the disorder can be gradual or sudden, and the severity of symptoms can vary over time.

Schizophrenia can also be perceived as an overblown imagination that would have become a reality. The main underlying symptom is called psychosis, and the presence of psychosis in an individual for generally six consecutive months can make a strong case of schizophrenia. The mind of a person with schizophrenia can be like the mind of someone "high" on cannabis. However, the schizophrenic patient would have no cannabis in their system.

Your Brain's General Mechanics

One must understand a few things about the mind to connect psychological symptoms that vary across the population to a drug of interest. Just as a car has

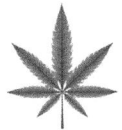

three primary functions: acceleration, braking, and turning, your mind works by doing three things: recall, understand, and apply information. Suppose the wiring and connections of your brain are impaired to cause a problem in any of those three areas. In that case, you will have a psychological problem.

On the other hand, **intellect** is the brain's ability to think or reason logically. It involves applying those three functions in a way that can be repeated with accuracy. In a way, what we refer to as intellect is like a manual for your brain; a process of using recall, understanding, and applying information to create a step-by-step process of reasoning and problem-solving. If any part of the brain structure (Can it work?), function (Does it work?), or intellect (How well does it work?) is compromised, there would be problems with learning and behaviour because that's how we observe the workings of the brain.

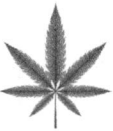

Intellect and Psychological Disorders

128

The ability to reason, problem-solve, and apply cognitive strategies can impact the experience and management of certain mental disorders. In the case of **obsessive-compulsive disorder** (OCD), an intact intellect can contribute to a better understanding of the irrationality or excessive nature of obsessions and compulsions, allowing individuals to challenge and resist them to some extent.

For individuals with a compromised intellect, the challenges in reasoning and cognitive flexibility may make it more difficult for them to challenge or override their obsessive thoughts and compulsive behaviours. In such cases, therapeutic interventions must address the specific symptoms and support the individual in developing strategies to compensate for cognitive deficits.

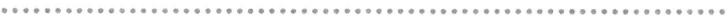

Treatment approaches for mental disorders often consider the individual's cognitive abilities and strengths. Cognitive-behavioural therapies, for instance, aim to modify maladaptive thoughts and behaviours through cognitive restructuring and developing coping mechanisms. The effectiveness of these therapies can be influenced by an individual's intellectual capacity to engage in the therapeutic process and apply learned strategies.

While individuals with higher intellect may have more cognitive resources to engage in therapy, treatment success also depends on factors such as the appropriateness of the treatment approach, the severity and chronicity of the disorder, individual motivation, support systems, and the presence of any comorbid conditions.

Cannabis and Hallucinations

Once cannabis establishes temporary residence in your brain, it can start playing with whatever is around—neurons and neurotransmitters, and interfere with normal structure and function. In the state of intoxication, cannabis can produce hallucinations, which is a normal effect. The problem comes when the state of being "high" is assumed to have passed, but the brain fails to reject persistent or recurring hallucinations and adopts the hallucinations as reality. At that point, the person will begin to exhibit symptoms of someone that is "high" while they aren't actually "high." This's the part where hallucinations are considered a disease because there's no stimulation of the symptoms, but the symptoms are present nonetheless.

129

This's most common when you consistently get high for days, weeks, months, or years and suddenly stop. While you stop using cannabis today, cannabis that had been stored over days, weeks, months, or years

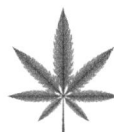

will start leaking out from the storage sites to enter your blood. When this happens, the hallucinations of cannabis intoxication can reoccur without euphoria— more about this later.

Some people still try to defend cannabis use as harmless when it comes to psychotic disorders. They state that other factors must be considered, like the possibility of cannabis being laced with other drugs. Another claim is that some people may not be "suitable candidates" for cannabis as they don't respond well to its consumption. Some have even argued that "people not smart enough to handle drugs" shouldn't take cannabis to the point of making it difficult for people that can handle the drug to acquire it.

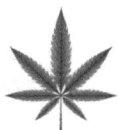

These arguments make sense to someone who is "high." How do we make that evaluation of someone's ability to handle cannabis before the damage is done? Should we take millions of lives and experiment with the long-term effects of cannabis consumption on their brains so that we can see if we can let it affect or help a million more? What's the worst that can happen if we study the effects of cannabis now before the widespread recreational use of cannabis? What's the worst that can happen if we allow the widespread use of recreational cannabis now and worry about the effects later? Which path is more ethical, economical, and sustainable for this and future generations—smoke now and worry later, or worry now and smoke later?

While it's true that illicit substances can sometimes be mixed with cannabis, it's essential to note that the discussion here primarily focuses on the effects of cannabis itself. Research has shown that cannabis use, even in its pure form, has been associated with an increased risk of developing psychotic symptoms and disorders, particularly in vulnerable individuals.

130

The argument about a patient's suitability to consume cannabis acknowledges that individual variations exist in how people react to cannabis, and some individuals may be more susceptible to the adverse effects. However, it's challenging to determine in advance who'll be negatively affected and who won't. Additionally, even if someone appears to handle cannabis well initially, the long-term effects on their mental health may still be a concern.

The idea of evaluating someone's ability to handle cannabis before any potential damage is done is a challenging proposition. It'd require comprehensive assessments of individuals' mental health and genetic predispositions, which isn't currently feasible on a widespread scale. When considering the potential effects of cannabis on mental health, it's crucial to prioritize the well-being and safety of individuals.

Conducting thorough scientific studies on the long-term effects of cannabis consumption can provide valuable insights into its potential risks and benefits. By gathering empirical evidence, we can make informed decisions about the possible consequences of widespread recreational cannabis use. This knowledge can guide regulations, education, and public health strategies to ensure the health and safety of current and future generations.

131

Choosing the path of studying the effects of cannabis now, before widespread recreational use, allows us to gather essential data and insights that can inform policy decisions and protective measures. By understanding the potential risks and implementing appropriate regulations, we can aim to minimize harm and promote responsible cannabis use for recreational purposes.

On the other hand, opting for widespread recreational use of cannabis without fully understanding its long-term effects may pose risks to public health. Without proper knowledge and regulations in place, there's a

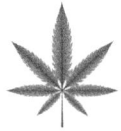

potential for increased negative consequences, particularly for vulnerable populations.

Regarding economic and sustainable outcomes, prioritizing research and understanding the effects of cannabis before widespread use can help minimize potential long-term costs associated with increased mental health issues and related healthcare expenses. It allows for evidence-based policies that strike a balance between individual freedoms and public health concerns.

Cannabis-induced Psychosis: The Protein-binding Effect

One plausible theory for the mechanism behind cannabis-induced psychosis lies in the drug's protein-binding affinity. When cannabis enters your body, it binds to proteins in your blood. As it crosses the blood-brain barrier, it can also attach to proteins in your brain, specifically neurotransmitters. These neurotransmitters are vital for normal brain function, as they play a crucial role in transmitting signals between nerve cells. However, when cannabis binds to these proteins, it interferes with their normal functioning, leading to a **pseudo-deficiency**. This means that the protein is still present in the body, but its availability for regular use is compromised because cannabis is holding onto it.

132

This protein-binding interference can negatively affect protein-based hormones in your blood, potentially contributing to various physiological effects. In your brain, where neurotransmitters are impacted, the altered signalling may disrupt normal brain processes, leading to changes in perception, cognition, and behaviour.

One possible consequence of this disruption is the development of psychotic symptoms, such as hallucinations and delusions, characteristic of conditions like

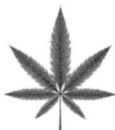

schizophrenia. The exact mechanisms by which cannabis-induced protein-binding affects brain function and leads to psychosis are still under investigation. Furthermore, cannabis use may also contribute to a loss of appetite, leading to reduced protein consumption. This creates an additional challenge as the body struggles to replenish the bound hormones and neurotransmitters, further exacerbating the adverse effects of cannabis' protein-binding capacity.

It's paramount to recognize that this's just one of several theories being explored to understand the link between cannabis and psychosis. The interaction of cannabis with your brain is incredibly intricate and influenced by various factors, including individual genetics, frequency and dosage of cannabis use, and pre-existing vulnerabilities.

The manifestation of psychotic symptoms and "odd behaviour" in some individuals after cannabis use underscores the need for continued research and a comprehensive understanding of this complex issue. Multiple scientific disciplines, including **neuroscience**, pharmacology, and **psychiatry**, are collaborating to shed light on these mechanisms and develop evidence-based approaches to address the potential risks associated with cannabis use.

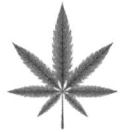

Man X was sitting on a tree branch he was cutting. He was not bothered at all, as he was focused on the task at hand. Man Y, walking past the tree, noticed this man sitting on the hanging part of the branch being cut, and he decided to offer a few words of advice. He told Man X to change how he was sitting and sit on the side of the branch closer to the tree trunk. Man Y told Man X that he feared that Man X would fall on the ground when the branch falls, and break his bones.

Man X ignored this and continued doing his job. A couple of minutes later, Man Y was returning past the same tree he had passed before and found Man X lying on the ground in agony. Man Y checked on Man X, who assured him he was fine despite the pain from falling from the tree. Before Man X could let Man Y go, he couldn't resist asking a burning question, which Man Y was willing to entertain. "You told me that I would fall when the branch falls, and look at me now. My question is, when am I going to die?" asked Man X.

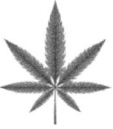

134

If you were Man Y, how would you have handled this inquiry?

All I Know Is I Want More

What is drug dependence?

The issue of cannabis dependence is a topic of ongoing debate and research. While some may argue that cannabis is not addictive, it's crucial to recognize that dependence on cannabis can occur. **Drug dependence** refers to the adaptive changes that occur in your brain as a result of repeated drug use, leading to **withdrawal symptoms** when the drug is discontinued or reduced.

Research has shown that a subset of individuals who use cannabis regularly can develop dependence, characterized by **cravings**, **tolerance** (needing more of the drug to achieve the same effects), and withdrawal symptoms when they try to quit or cut down their use. These withdrawal symptoms may include **irritability**, sleep difficulties, anxiety, and changes in appetite.

It's worth noting that the likelihood of developing cannabis dependence can vary among individuals. Some individuals may be more susceptible to developing cannabis dependence than others.

135

While the level of cannabis dependence may differ from substances like alcohol, **nicotine**, or **cocaine**, it's essential to recognize that dependence can still occur and can significantly impact your life and well-being. It's crucial to approach cannabis use cautiously and be aware of the potential risks and consequences of regular and heavy use.

Physical dependence

Drug dependence is typically grouped into **physical dependence** and **psychological dependence**. Physical dependence is a condition that occurs when your body adapts to the presence of a specific substance,

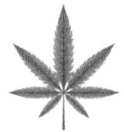

and its normal functioning becomes reliant on the continued use of that substance. When you develop physical dependence, your body adjusts its normal functioning to accommodate that substance.

Regular and prolonged use of certain drugs, such as opioids, sedatives, and alcohol, can lead to physical dependence. In these cases, your body becomes accustomed to the effects of the drug and adapts its functioning accordingly. When the drug is abruptly reduced or discontinued, your body will experience withdrawal symptoms as it readjusts to functioning without the substance.

Withdrawal symptoms can manifest as physical, emotional, and psychological effects. Physical symptoms may include **tremors**, sweating, nausea, headaches, **muscle aches**, and changes in appetite. Emotional and psychological symptoms can include anxiety, depression, irritability, **restlessness**, and difficulty concentrating.

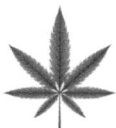

136

Withdrawal symptoms can be an exaggerated physiological response that occurs when you stop using a substance to which you have become physically dependent. The symptoms often reflect the opposite effects of the drug you were using.

For example, if a drug causes constipation, your body may become accustomed to that effect. When you stop or significantly reduce your consumption of the drug, your body's natural bowel function can rebound, leading to **diarrhea**.

The severity of withdrawal symptoms can vary depending on several factors, including the specific substance, the duration and intensity of use, and individual differences. In some cases, withdrawal symptoms can be quite severe and may even pose risks to your health and well-being. This's especially true for substances such as alcohol, opioids, and benzodiazepines.

It's important to note that physical dependence is different from **addiction**, although the two terms are sometimes used interchangeably. Addiction involves a complex interplay of physical, psychological, and behavioural factors, and it's characterized by compulsive drug-seeking behaviour and the inability to control drug use despite negative consequences. On the other hand, physical dependence primarily refers to the physiological changes that occur in response to continued drug exposure.

Case in point: alcohol is a substance that depresses or slows down your brain activity. When you consume alcohol over a prolonged period, your body adjusts to the presence of alcohol and adapts its normal functioning accordingly. Your brain becomes accustomed to the depressive effects of alcohol, which leads to decreased brain activity.

137

Suppose you abruptly stop drinking or significantly reduce your alcohol intake. In that case, your brain will no longer have the suppressive effects of alcohol. This sudden change can result in a rebound effect, causing your brain to become overactive. This overactivity can manifest as alcohol withdrawal symptoms.

Alcohol withdrawal symptoms can range from mild to severe and typically include physical, emotional, and psychological symptoms. These symptoms may include tremors, sweating, nausea, anxiety, restlessness, insomnia, irritability, increased heart rate, and seizures or **delirium tremens** in severe cases.

The severity and duration of alcohol withdrawal symptoms can vary depending on factors such as the amount and duration of alcohol use, individual differences, and previous experiences with with-

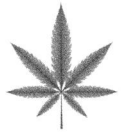

drawal. It's worth noting that alcohol withdrawal can be a potentially dangerous condition, especially in severe cases, and may require medical supervision and intervention.

Think of yourself sitting on a spring that is initially five metres high. The more you drink, the more the spring is compressed. When you get drunk once, that's equivalent to a ten-centimetre compression on that five-metre spring. Getting sober the following day is like the spring returning to its normal five-metre height. If you become a regular drinker, you compress that spring more and more until you reach the maximum compression of, say, three metres.

Now, imagine suddenly releasing the pressure on that spring after so much compression for a long time. In which case do you think you'll be shot higher into the air by the spring—the case where you only compress the spring by ten centimetres or the case where you compress the spring by three metres? In the first case of a ten-centimetre compression, you get drunk only one night after a few weeks of no alcohol consumption. The next day, your hangover equals how much space the spring will give you if you release the pressure. The typical symptoms of this hangover are headache, nausea, and irritability.

On the other extreme is the case of a three-metre spring compression. The more you compress the spring, the larger the spring force that'll lead to a higher launch into the air if the pressure on the spring is relieved. This scenario depicts a chronic alcoholic sitting on a spring for an extended period while it was compressed to three metres. The height of the launch represents the effects of suddenly stopping alcohol consumption; **alcohol withdrawal**. The symptoms of alcohol withdrawal were mentioned earlier.

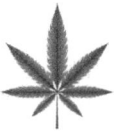

Psychological dependence

While some drugs may not lead to significant physical withdrawal symptoms upon discontinuation, they can still result in intense cravings and psychological dependence. Psychological dependence refers to the emotional and psychological need for a substance, even in the face of negative consequences.

In psychological dependence, you may experience a strong desire or craving to use the substance, which can be challenging to control. You may feel that you need the substance to cope with certain emotions, to feel pleasure, or to function in your daily life. This psychological need can drive compulsive drug-seeking behaviours, even when you know the harmful effects and negative consequences of substance use.

Psychological dependence can profoundly impact your thoughts, emotions, and behaviours. It can lead to a loss of control over drug use, difficulties in managing relationships and responsibilities, and a preoccupation with obtaining and using the substance. Over time, psychological dependence can significantly impair your overall well-being and quality of life.

It's vital to recognize that psychological dependence can occur independently of physical dependence or addiction. While physical dependence involves physiological changes in your body in response to the drug, psychological dependence is primarily driven by emotional and psychological factors.

Psychological dependence on a drug can lead to various challenges and negative consequences in your life. The cravings and strong urges to use the drug can be challenging to resist, and you may feel a sense of discomfort or distress when you are unable to fulfill those cravings.

The impact of psychological dependence extends beyond your internal experiences. It can affect your re-

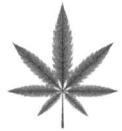

139

lationships, work or school performance, and overall functioning in daily life. The preoccupation with obtaining and using the substance can lead to strained relationships with family, friends, and colleagues. It may also result in decreased productivity, absenteeism, or poor academic performance.

Financial difficulties can arise due to excessive spending on the substance or legal consequences if the drug use leads to illegal activities. You may find it challenging to maintain stability in your personal and professional life, leading to a cycle of negative outcomes and further reinforcing the dependence.

The development of psychological dependence is a complex process influenced by various factors. Genetics can play a role in your vulnerability to developing dependence on certain substances. Environmental factors, such as exposure to drug use in your surroundings or substance availability, can also contribute to psychological dependence.

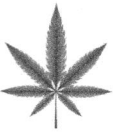

140

Personal life experiences, including trauma, stress, or certain mental health conditions, can increase your risk of developing dependence as you may turn to drugs as a coping mechanism. The interplay between **brain chemistry** and substance use is another critical factor. Prolonged drug use can lead to changes in your **brain's reward system**, reinforcing the desire to continue using the substance.

Fear of withdrawal symptoms can also contribute to the maintenance of psychological dependence. You may continue using the substance to avoid or alleviate the discomfort that arises when you attempt to quit or reduce its use.

It's worth noting that psychological dependence often coexists with physical dependence. The combination of psychological and physical dependence can create a powerful cycle of addiction, making it challenging to break free from substance use or abuse.

Think of your relationship with food. You eat when you're hungry, angry, upset, or just bored. Hunger is the physical sensation that signals your body's need for nourishment and sustenance. It's a biological response that occurs when your body requires energy and nutrients. That's why you can devour anything, even food you typically dislike when you're starving.

However, sometimes you don't really feel the physical need to consume food, but feel the need to have something specific. You can eat dinner and feel physically full, but still think about eating that chocolate cake you have thought about all day. This psychological need to eat something specific is called appetite, which is why we routinely talk about having an appetite for something specific.

On the other hand, appetite is more related to the psychological aspect of wanting to eat. It is influenced by factors such as emotions, memories, cultural influences, and personal preferences. The physical need for food doesn't solely drive appetite but rather the desire to consume specific foods that are appealing or satisfying to you.

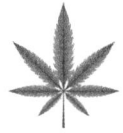

141

Cravings take appetite to another level. They're intense desires for specific foods, often accompanied by vivid thoughts and images of the desired food. Cravings can be triggered by various factors, including exposure to certain smells or sights, emotional states, or even just the thought of a particular food. When cravings occur, people may experience physiological responses like excessive swallowing, teeth grinding, an uncontrollable grin, or increased breathing, among others.

Cravings can be powerful and lead individuals to go to great lengths to satisfy them. It's not uncommon for people to make impulsive decisions, change their plans, or engage in behaviours they wouldn't typically do in order to fulfill their cravings. People may jump through hoops to satisfy that craving, from heading to a drive-thru a few hours before dawn to chasing a food truck at full speed.

Things get slightly more intense when this craving is for a specific drug. A very common drug for this kind of dependence is nicotine. Do you want to see anger? Just hide a pack of cigarettes from someone heavily dependent on nicotine. Instead of chasing a truck, some people will be willing to crawl on broken glass with their tongues to reach for the burning stub of a cigarette thrown away by a fellow smoker.

Nicotine is a highly addictive substance found in to-bacco products, and it can lead to a strong psycholog-ical dependence in individuals who use it regularly. Psychological dependence on nicotine is character-ized by intense cravings for nicotine and a compel-ling desire to use tobacco products. These cravings can be triggered by various cues, such as certain sit-uations, emotions, or even the sight or smell of cig-arettes. The desire to satisfy these cravings can be so powerful that some individuals may go to great lengths to obtain nicotine.

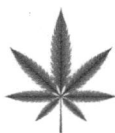

142

The cravings experienced in psychological depen-dence on nicotine can be overwhelming and challeng-ing to resist. They can lead to a sense of loss of control over one's behaviour and an intense preoccupation with obtaining and using nicotine.

Caffeine is another example of a substance that can lead to both physical and psychological dependence. Many individuals rely on caffeine, commonly found in coffee, tea, energy drinks, and other beverages, to help them stay alert and combat fatigue.

Regularly consuming caffeine makes your body ac-customed to its presence, leading to physical depen-dence. Abruptly stopping or significantly reducing caffeine intake can result in withdrawal symptoms, typically occurring within one to five days after the last cup of coffee. Common withdrawal symptoms include headaches that may not respond to over-the-counter pain relievers, persistent nervousness, irritability, fatigue, and difficulty concentrating.

In addition to physical dependence, caffeine can also trigger psychological dependence. This psychological aspect is characterized by a strong desire or craving for the taste, ritual, or experience associated with caffeine consumption. Some individuals may feel strongly attached to their daily coffee or the routine of brewing and enjoying a cup.

It's important to note that the severity and duration of caffeine withdrawal symptoms can vary among individuals. Factors such as the amount of caffeine consumed, the frequency of use, and individual differences in metabolism can influence the withdrawal experience.

Social dependence

143

There's a third kind of dependence that can neither be described as cravings nor withdrawal symptoms. This's when people think the drug amplifies their personality, creativity, concentration, or confidence. It's not necessarily the effect of the drug on the brain that people will appreciate. Instead, that boost in confidence makes it easier for them to be social, stand up for themselves, or have faith in themselves more. When that person doesn't take their dose of the drug, they'll become the exact opposite of the way they are under the influence of the drug. If the drug helps them talk to girls, they'll be unable to even mutter a word to a girl as long as they believe they don't have that drug in their system. This isn't enough to call this any kind of dependence because if you give some of these people a sugar pill and tell them it'll make them talk to girls with confidence, there's a high likelihood that the sugar pill will work if they believe for once

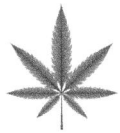

that it will. This's called a placebo effect. It's unlikely that you'll be able to use a **placebo effect** to help someone with cravings for cocaine or someone undergoing alcohol withdrawal.

Sometimes, you may believe a particular drug enhances your personality traits, creativity, concentration, or confidence. This psychological dependence is driven by the perceived positive effects of the drug on your mental state or performance.

In such situations, you may feel that you need the drug to access those enhanced qualities or capabilities. Your confidence or belief in your abilities may be closely tied to the drug's influence on your mindset. This can create a psychological reliance on the drug to reproduce those desired effects in specific situations or contexts.

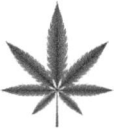

144

It's worth noting that the placebo effect can play a role in the psychological dependence of certain substances. Placebos are inert substances or treatments with no physiological effect, but their administration can lead to perceived improvements or relief due to your belief in their efficacy. Placebo effects can be influenced by various factors, including your expectations, conditioning, and the context in which the placebo is administered.

Ultimately, the complexities of dependence, including physical, psychological, and placebo effects, highlight the multifaceted nature of human responses to drugs. Understanding these factors can contribute to more comprehensive approaches to supporting individuals who may be struggling with substance use issues.

The concept of "social dependence" refers to the perceived need for a substance to facilitate social interactions or enhance certain qualities or abilities. This social dependence can stem from the belief that the drug makes the person more intelligent, sexier, creative, or socially adept.

However, it's important to distinguish between the subjective experiences or perceived benefits individuals may associate with drug use and the actual cognitive or intellectual enhancement that drugs can provide. While some individuals may feel that drugs allow them to function at a level comparable to others, it's essential to consider the potential risks and limitations of drug use.

Drugs don't inherently make a person smarter. Intellectual capacities and problem-solving abilities are influenced by a wide range of factors, including genetics, education, environment, and cognitive skills that go beyond the influence of drugs.

However, it's worth acknowledging that some individuals may rely on certain medications, such as those prescribed for anxiety or stress, to manage symptoms that may otherwise hinder their cognitive functioning. These medications can alleviate underlying psychological tension and help individuals function optimally by reducing impairments caused by anxiety or stress.

145

In any case, it's vital to approach drug use and its perceived benefits with caution and critical thinking. Substance use should be carefully evaluated based on individual circumstances, potential risks, and the guidance of healthcare professionals.

Cannabis Dependence

Understanding the potential for physical dependence on cannabis requires us to delve into its pharmacology and physiology of the human body. While there hasn't been a specific scientific study addressing this question, we can explore relevant information to shed light on the topic.

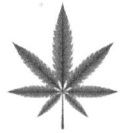

First, let's consider the pharmacological properties of cannabis. When you consume cannabis, THC enters your bloodstream and is distributed throughout your body. Due to its fat-soluble nature, THC can readily penetrate fatty tissues, including your brain, where it exerts its effects.

To better grasp the implications of cannabis storage and breakdown, you need to understand your body's handling of the drug. Once THC enters your body, it undergoes various metabolic processes. The liver plays a crucial role in metabolizing THC, breaking it down into metabolites that can be eliminated from your body. However, some THC and its metabolites can be stored in fatty tissues for extended periods.

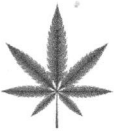

This storage in fatty tissues has implications for potential physical dependence. While THC itself isn't considered physically addictive in the same way as substances like opioids or alcohol, the prolonged presence of THC and its metabolites in fatty tissues can lead to a phenomenon known as **drug reservoirs**. These reservoirs can slowly release THC back into the bloodstream over time, even after cannabis use has ceased.

146

The release of THC from these reservoirs can potentially trigger a reactivation of the drug's effects, which may contribute to cravings or a desire to use cannabis again. It's important to note that these cravings may have a psychological component, as individuals associate the effects of cannabis with certain experiences or feelings.

It's worth emphasizing that physical dependence on cannabis, if it occurs, is generally considered milder compared to substances like opioids or alcohol. Withdrawal symptoms associated with cannabis cessation, if present at all, are typically mild and transient, including irritability, insomnia, and changes in appetite.

These symptoms are generally far less severe than those observed with substances known to cause significant physical dependence.

While scientific studies specifically examining physical dependence on cannabis are limited, the existing evidence suggests that physical dependence development is less pronounced than other substances. However, individual responses to cannabis can vary, and some individuals may experience stronger cravings or difficulties discontinuing use.

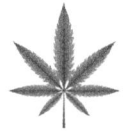

147

A single mother of two knew she wouldn't be home on time to make dinner for her sons. She called home and told the older son to cook for his younger brother as she was running late. The older brother assured her he would take good care of his little brother.

The older brother explained the situation to his brother and gave him two options. He said, "I could make dinner for you, or order pizza." The little brother lit up with joy as he heard the word pizza. He yelled, "Pizza!"

Pizza was ordered, and dinner was done within an hour. When the mother got home, she asked where to find the cooked food. The younger brother quickly answered, "Sorry, Mom, we ate it all." She knew her sons all too well and didn't buy this for once. She turned to the older son and asked, "You bought pizza, didn't you?" She didn't even give the son time to answer, and she called him irresponsible.

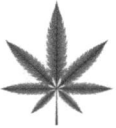

148

The older brother asked his younger brother what he wanted and got him exactly that. Was the brother irresponsible, or was he just acting democratically?

It's A Drug, It's A Crime, It's A Cure!

The Basics of Cannabis Metabolism

When you consume cannabis, it enters your bloodstream. Once in your bloodstream, THC can bind to cannabinoid receptors in your brain, leading to the euphoric and relaxing sensations commonly associated with cannabis use.

After entering your bloodstream, THC undergoes **metabolism** in your liver. The liver breaks down THC into **metabolites**, such as **11-hydroxy-THC** and **THC-COOH**, through a series of reactions involving specific liver enzymes. These metabolites are then eliminated from your body through urine and feces.

It's important to note that the metabolism and elimination of cannabis and its metabolites can vary among individuals. Factors such as frequency and dose of cannabis use, individual metabolism, and other physiological factors can influence how long THC and its metabolites remain detectable in your body.

149

As mentioned earlier, some of the consumed cannabis can also bind to hormones and neurotransmitters or be stored in fatty tissues throughout your body. This storage in fatty tissues can gradually release THC back into your bloodstream over time, which may contribute to its prolonged effects and potential to reactivate drug effects.

It's worth mentioning that the presence of THC in fatty tissues can also result in positive drug tests for cannabis, even after a considerable amount of time has passed since the last use. Drug tests typically detect THC-COOH, one of the metabolites of THC, in urine or other bodily fluids.

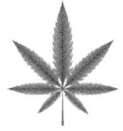

While the process of metabolism and elimination helps remove cannabis and its metabolites from your body, it's important to note that the effects of cannabis can vary depending on factors such as the strain, potency, and method of consumption. Additionally, individual responses to cannabis can differ, and some individuals may experience a range of effects beyond relaxation or pain relief.

Understanding the **pharmacokinetics** of cannabis, including its absorption, distribution, metabolism, and elimination, helps us comprehend how the drug interacts with your body and how it may potentially lead to dependence or other effects.

The effect of frequent consumption

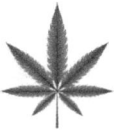

150

If you consume more cannabis and more frequently, proteins in your blood where cannabis initially binds will eventually get overwhelmed by the drug. Think of your blood with only ten cannabis molecules that can interact with proteins—and you have twenty molecules of proteins. Ten molecules of cannabis will bind to ten protein molecules. This leaves ten protein molecules unbound, but that would be 50% fewer active proteins. Less active proteins in your blood may affect some of your metabolic processes depending on the proteins taken out of circulation. Thus, it could be dangerous for large amounts of cannabis to be in the blood at the same time. However, your body will still try to find ways to make cannabis less toxic to your body.

Proteins play vital roles in various metabolic processes, including **enzyme activities**, transport of substances, and immune responses. When cannabis molecules bind to proteins, it can alter their normal functioning and potentially interfere with these essential processes.

Remember that cannabis is a fat-soluble drug, meaning it likes to interact with fatty substances? If your blood can only handle thirty molecules of cannabis, after the first ten cannabis molecules bind to the ten proteins, twenty cannabis molecules will stay in your blood to make you see music, hear colours, and give you the munchies. At the same time, the rest of the cannabis will have to be stored elsewhere. When you consume a lot of cannabis and exceed the thirty-molecule threshold, the rest of the cannabis you consume will start getting stored in other mostly fatty tissues like your brain, bone marrow, and muscle. Without a doubt, cannabis can also be kept in the fat around your belly, thighs, arms, or even testicles.

It's important to note that the storage of cannabis in fatty tissues is a natural process that occurs with many fat-soluble substances. The stored cannabis can be gradually released back into your bloodstream over time, prolonging its effects on your body.

It's worth mentioning that the accumulation of cannabis in fatty tissues can have implications for drug testing. Even after the acute effects of cannabis have worn off, **residual cannabis metabolites** can be detected in bodily fluids, such as urine or hair, due to the release from fat stores. This's why cannabis can be detected in drug tests for an extended period after use.

As blood is pumped throughout your body to supply nutrients, it also passes through your liver. Your liver is your body's center for detoxification. This's where things that may harm your body are broken down and sent for elimination. Your liver also contains certain enzymes to break down certain drugs and biochemicals.

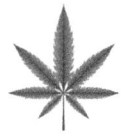

151

Cannabis and Enzyme Induction

Suppose your liver uses enzyme A to break down cannabis. In that case, when there's too much cannabis in your body than it can handle, your liver will make more enzyme A to keep up with breaking down the excess cannabis. This increased enzyme production is known as **enzyme induction**. This process aims to enhance the breakdown and elimination of cannabis from your body.

However, an unintended consequence of enzyme induction is that it can affect the metabolism of other drugs that utilize the same enzymes. Let's consider drug B, which is typically broken down by enzyme A. When enzyme A is induced by cannabis, it becomes more abundant in your liver and can metabolize drug B at an accelerated rate. This can result in drug B being broken down more quickly than intended, leading to reduced effectiveness or a shorter duration of action.

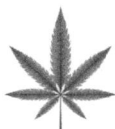

152

This phenomenon is known as **drug-drug interactions**, where one drug influences the metabolism or effects of another drug. Drug-drug interactions can occur with various medications, not just cannabis.

The specific drug-drug interactions involving cannabis and other substances will depend on the particular drugs involved, their metabolic pathways, and individual variations in enzyme activity. Quite often, people wake up during surgery because the anesthesia wears out too quickly due to this effect. The common causes of this effect are not limited to frequent alcohol and tobacco use.

The Effect of Alcohol on OCPs

Alcohol consumption can lead to an induction of liver enzymes responsible for breaking down alcohol, which can also affect the metabolism of other drugs, including OCPs. In this scenario, when a young woman drinks alcohol, her liver produces more enzymes to metabolize the alcohol. These same enzymes are involved in breaking down the hormones present in OCPs. As a result, the increased enzyme activity from drinking alcohol can accelerate the metabolism of OCPs, causing them to be eliminated from her body more rapidly than expected.

Suppose OCPs are metabolized and eliminated too quickly. In that case, their concentration in her blood may fall below the adequate level required for contraception. This reduced concentration of OCPs can compromise their contraceptive effectiveness and increase the risk of pregnancy.

From the moment anything enters your body, it encounters several defence mechanisms used by your body to keep infections and toxins away. If that toxin or chemical surpasses all those defences and reaches your blood, your liver will be your last line of defence. The human liver is the most complicated organ in the human body when it comes to functionality. Your liver has nearly a dozen essential functions to help your body achieve optimal health. One of these many functions is the ability to make toxins and chemicals benign to your body by applying various enzymes in biochemical reactions.

153

All in all, enzymes are of different kinds and affect different drugs differently. Some people have some enzymes but not others. Inasmuch as we all appear different on the outside, we're also functionally different on the inside.

The Importance of Your Liver in Drug Metabolism

Your liver is crucial to your body's defence mechanisms and overall health. It's involved in numerous functions, including detoxifying and metabolizing

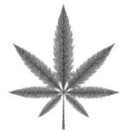

drugs and toxins. Enzymes, special proteins produced by your liver, facilitate the chemical reactions that break down and transform drugs and toxins in your body. These enzymes can modify the structure of substances, making them less harmful or facilitating their elimination from your body.

Different enzymes in your liver have specific roles in metabolizing different drugs and toxins. The activity and levels of these enzymes can vary among individuals. Some people may have higher levels of certain enzymes, while others may have lower levels or may lack specific enzymes altogether. This individual variation in enzyme activity can affect how drugs are processed and eliminated from your body.

For example, certain drugs require specific enzymes for their metabolism. If you lack the necessary enzyme, the drug may not be broken down effectively, leading to a buildup of the drug in your body and potentially causing adverse effects. On the other hand, if you have higher levels of a particular enzyme, the drug may be metabolized more rapidly, resulting in reduced effectiveness.

This interplay between enzymes and drugs is vital in personalized medicine and understanding how individuals may respond differently to medications. Genetic factors can influence enzyme activity, and ongoing research is focused on understanding these variations to optimize drug therapy and minimize adverse effects.

It's worth noting that the complex nature of drug metabolism and enzyme interactions means that drug interactions can be unpredictable and vary from person to person.

The Metabolism of Alcohol

When you start drinking alcohol, you'll most likely not become drunk after the first couple of sips. If you do

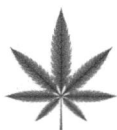

get drunk with only a couple of sips, you probably shouldn't be consuming alcohol in the first place.

When you consume alcohol, your liver enzymes break it down and eliminate it from your body. Initially, the enzymes can handle the alcohol relatively steadily, allowing your body to process it efficiently. However, as you continue to drink alcohol, especially in larger quantities, the rate at which your liver enzymes can metabolize the alcohol may become overwhelmed. This can result in a buildup of alcohol in your bloodstream, making its effects more pronounced and affecting various body processes.

The accumulation of alcohol in your blood can impair cognitive function, motor skills, and coordination. It can also affect other bodily functions such as digestion, hormone regulation, and the functioning of the nervous system. Additionally, prolonged or excessive alcohol consumption can have serious health consequences, including liver damage, cardiovascular problems, and an increased risk of developing certain types of cancer.

155

It's important to remember that everyone's tolerance to alcohol can vary based on factors such as body weight, metabolism, and individual differences in liver enzyme activity.

Alcohol tolerance and interaction with other drugs

Regular alcohol consumption can lead to your body's adaptation, including the liver, to better metabolize alcohol. This adaptation involves the increased production of enzymes responsible for breaking down alcohol, which allows your body to process alcohol more efficiently over time. As a result, individuals who regularly drink alcohol may develop a higher tolerance, requiring larger amounts of alcohol to experience the same effects they initially felt with smaller quantities.

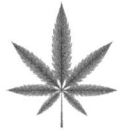

However, this increased enzyme activity can also impact the breakdown of other substances in your body, including medications like OCPs and antidepressants. The enzymes that break down alcohol may also break down these medications faster, potentially reducing their effectiveness or altering their intended effects. This can have important implications for individuals who rely on these medications. It's important to note that the interactions between alcohol and medications can vary depending on the specific drug and individual factors.

Think about it. If you have a hundred enzymes to break down alcohol when you have your very first beer, this number can increase to a hundred thousand to keep up with your drinking. If one OCP worked for you before your first drink at sixteen years of age with only a hundred enzymes to break it down, do you think one OCP will stand a chance once it has a hundred thousand enzymes to break it down? The answer is no, and it's why some women end up getting pregnant despite regularly taking their pills as prescribed. The point is that stimulating enzymes by one drug can lead to the inefficiency of another drug.

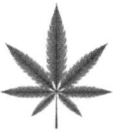

Cannabis Liver Metabolism

Cannabis also interacts with enzymes in your liver, specifically the **cytochrome P450** enzymes, which are responsible for metabolizing a wide range of substances, including certain drugs. The active compounds in cannabis, such as THC, can interact with these enzymes and potentially impact the metabolism of drugs that are broken down by the same enzymes.

This interaction can affect the levels of medications in your body, either increasing or decreasing their concentration, which may influence their effectiveness or lead to unexpected side effects. Therefore, it's crucial to inform your healthcare provider about your cannabis use to ensure they can provide appropriate guidance and monitor your treatment accordingly.

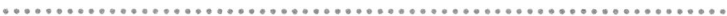

Liver Enzymes and Drug Inhibition

In addition to stimulating enzymes, inhibiting enzymes by certain drugs can also significantly affect the metabolism of other drugs in your body. When drug A inhibits the activity of enzyme B responsible for metabolizing another drug B, it can lead to an accumulation of drug B in your body.

This can have various consequences. Firstly, the increased concentration of the drug may cause it to reach higher than intended levels, potentially leading to adverse effects or toxicity. Secondly, suppose the inhibited enzyme B is responsible for converting drug B into its active form. In that case, the reduced metabolism can result in decreased therapeutic efficacy.

It's important to note that drug interactions can be complex and depend on various factors such as the specific drugs involved, individual genetic differences, dosage, and duration of use.

Example of Drug Interaction

157

An excellent example is of these two common medications: **erythromycin** (an **antibiotic**) and **warfarin** (an **anticoagulant**). Imagine receiving long-term **anticoagulation** treatment with warfarin to prevent blood clots, and you develop an infection. Erythromycin inhibits some liver enzymes, and these same liver enzymes are responsible for breaking down warfarin. Problem: how can your liver break down warfarin now that warfarin's enzymes have been put out of play by erythromycin?

When enzymes that break down warfarin are inhibited, the clearance of warfarin from your body slows down. This means that warfarin remains in your bloodstream longer, leading to higher drug levels and a prolonged anticoagulant effect. This can increase the risk of bleeding because warfarin's blood-thinning properties are amplified.
As long as you continue to take warfarin, excess warfa-

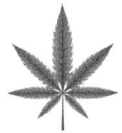

rin will accumulate in your blood, impeding your ability to form clots. This includes clots your body needs to stop spontaneous bleeding in your nose, stomach, bladder, and even your lungs due to minor chemical or physical trauma in small blood vessels. This drug interaction can lead to excessive bleeding internally or externally. Death can result if this bleeding isn't treated, or if these medications aren't stopped. While this was discovered in the eighties, you can imagine how many people had to die before the effect of this drug interaction was observed.

In the past, it took time and observation to identify these types of drug interactions and understand their consequences. Clinical experience, post-marketing surveillance, and research studies have contributed to our current understanding of drug interactions and their associated risks. As a result, healthcare professionals now have access to information that can help them anticipate potential interactions and take appropriate measures to ensure patient safety.

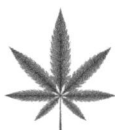

158

However, it's crucial to recognize that drug interactions can still occur. New interactions may be discovered as more medications and therapies are developed. Continued vigilance and communication between healthcare providers and patients are essential to effectively detect and manage these interactions.

The medical community strives to improve drug safety by researching, monitoring adverse events, and updating prescribing guidelines. This ongoing effort helps identify and mitigate potential risks associated with drug interactions, ultimately aiming to improve patient outcomes and minimize harm.

Cannabis and Drug Interaction

The metabolism of cannabis and the specific enzymes involved in its breakdown are still not fully understood. This lack of knowledge contributes to the variability in the effects of cannabis observed among different individuals. How your body processes and responds to cannabis can be influenced by various factors, including genetics, liver function, and interactions with other medications or substances.

The enzymes responsible for breaking down cannabis in the liver are part of cytochrome P450 enzymes. These enzymes are crucial in metabolizing a wide range of drugs and substances in your body. However, the specific enzymes involved in cannabis metabolism have not been definitively identified.

Furthermore, the metabolism of cannabis can be influenced by other drugs that interact with the same liver enzymes. For example, taking another medication that inhibits these enzymes may lead to higher levels of cannabis in your body and potentially intensified effects. On the other hand, if a drug induces the activity of these enzymes, it may result in faster breakdown of cannabis and potentially reduced effects.

The individual variations in enzyme activity, genetic factors, and drug interactions contribute to the unique responses people have to cannabis. It highlights the importance of considering these factors when using cannabis or when using other medications alongside cannabis.

159

Enzyme Variations Among Different Populations

Enzyme variations among different populations can significantly impact how substances, including alcohol, are metabolized in your body. People of Asian heritage and women, in general, may have lower levels of **alcohol dehydrogenase** enzymes, which are responsible for breaking down alcohol. As a result, they may experience a faster buildup of alcohol in their bloodstream, leading to quicker intoxication compared to other individuals.

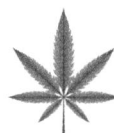

Similarly, when it comes to cannabis metabolism, there's a possibility of interindividual differences based on enzyme activity and genetic factors. While the specific enzymes involved in cannabis metabolism aren't yet well characterized, it's plausible that variations in these enzymes can influence how cannabis is processed in your body.

Moreover, cannabis may also interact with enzymes involved in the metabolism of other drugs, potentially affecting their efficacy and toxicity. This highlights the importance of considering potential drug interactions and individual variations when using cannabis in conjunction with other medications.

The Effect of Muscle and Fat on cannabis distribution

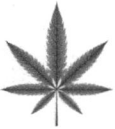

Cannabis, a fat-soluble drug, accumulates in fatty tissues such as the brain, muscle, and bone marrow. This can lead to variations in the amount of cannabis stored among different individuals, particularly considering differences in body composition.

While brain size is relatively consistent among individuals, variations in muscle and fat content can impact the storage capacity of cannabis. For instance, if we consider a group of people who regularly use cannabis over some time, individuals with lower fat content may have a relatively lower amount of cannabis stored compared to individuals with higher fat content.

It's worth noting that, on average, women tend to have more body fat than men. Consequently, women may have a higher potential to store cannabis in their bodies compared to men of the same weight. However, it's crucial to recognize that individual variations exist within both genders, and factors such as metabolism, genetics, and frequency of use can also contribute to the distribution and storage of cannabis in your body.

Understanding these variations in cannabis storage can have implications for the effects and potential risks associated with long-term cannabis use. It highlights the need to consider individual factors and body composition when assessing the impact of cannabis on different individuals.

Effect of Hormonal Difference on Cannabis Efficacy

Hormonal differences between genders can contribute to variations in body composition and fat distribution. Testosterone, which is more predominant in men, promotes muscle growth and tends to result in lower fat storage compared to estrogen, which is more predominant in women and promotes fat storage. Breasts are primarily composed of fatty tissue, which can further contribute to the differences in fat storage capacity between men and women.

Beyond gender differences, several other factors can influence the storage capacity of cannabis within individuals of the same gender. These factors include genetics, age, metabolism, overall body composition, and lifestyle habits such as diet and exercise. All these factors can play a role in the amount of fatty tissue available for cannabis storage. They may contribute to variations in the effects and risks associated with long-term cannabis use.

Body mass index (BMI) can play a role in the storage capacity of cannabis in your body. Generally, individuals with higher BMIs tend to have a larger overall body size, including a higher proportion of fatty tissue. Since cannabis is a fat-soluble drug, it's more likely to accumulate and be stored in the fatty tissues of individuals with higher BMIs compared to those with lower BMIs.

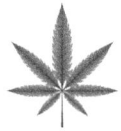

161

Chronic Cannabis Use, Storage, Release from Storage, and Testing

In chronic cannabis use, your body may develop tolerance, leading to a higher dose requirement to achieve the same level of intoxication. This tolerance can result from various factors, including increased liver enzyme activity and changes in the sensitivity of cannabinoid receptors in your brain.

When the concentration of cannabis in your blood decreases, stored THC in fatty tissues can be gradually released back into your bloodstream. The rate of release and the duration of detectability can be influenced by factors such as body fat percentage, metabolism, frequency of use, and other individual characteristics.

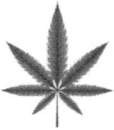

162

For heavy cannabis users, THC can potentially be detected in urine for up to several weeks after the last use, as THC metabolites are excreted in the urine. Blood and saliva tests generally have a shorter detection window, typically ranging from a few hours to a few days after use, depending on the frequency and amount of recent cannabis consumption. Hair tests have a longer detection window and can detect cannabis use over several months. However, hair tests are less commonly used due to their expense and complexity.

Unlike alcohol, which has established guidelines for **blood alcohol concentration** (BAC) and corresponding levels of intoxication, there're currently no standardized guidelines for **blood cannabis levels** and intoxication. The effects of cannabis and the corresponding THC metabolites can vary widely among individuals due to factors such as tolerance, frequency and amount of use, method of consumption, and individual sensitivity.

With chronic cannabis use and increased liver enzyme activity, higher doses of cannabis may be required to achieve the desired level of intoxication.
This phenomenon is known as **tolerance**. However,
it's important to note that tolerance to the subjective effects of cannabis doesn't necessarily indicate
an absence of impairment or risk, particularly when
engaging in activities that require cognitive or motor skills, such as driving.

The release of stored cannabis from fatty tissues and
fluctuations in blood cannabis levels can be influenced
by various factors, including individual metabolism,
body fat percentage, and other drugs. Drug interactions, especially with fat-soluble drugs, can potentially
displace cannabis from blood proteins and fatty tissues, leading to increased concentrations of cannabis
in your bloodstream.

The complex nature of cannabis metabolism and its
interactions with other substances make it challenging to predict and determine precise blood cannabis
levels and their corresponding effects on intoxication.

163

Fat is a form of energy, and in times of stress or
hunger, this fat is broken down to release its energy. In addition, this fat will also release stored
cannabis into your system. This can be caused by
starvation or any of the stress hormones: testosterone, cortisol, growth hormone, glucagon, and
epinephrine/norepinephrine.
Testosterone can be induced by intense physical activities, cortisol by any stress, glucagon by starvation,
and the last one is commonly induced by smoking cigarettes. Other reasons ranging from infection to quit-
ting the drug, can all result in unpredictable levels of
cannabis in your blood at any given time.
Suppose you're a regular cannabis user, and you suddenly stop smoking. In that case, cannabis will slowly

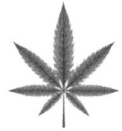

leak out of your fatty tissues at the speed of a chameleon over weeks to months. You'll likely feel normal with no withdrawal signs. However, when you induce the release of any stress hormones, cannabis will leak out of your fatty tissues at the speed of a cheater. You may experience transient effects that may resemble being under the influence of cannabis.

Imagine going a week without puffing the magic dragon, then suddenly feeling like you're high after smoking a cigarette. While most won't notice the difference in themselves, those around them will undoubtedly ask, "What's going on?" These are the withdrawal effects of cannabis that are very difficult to describe or explain, but this's typically the underlying mechanism. The symptoms are also too complicated to fit the description of physical dependence.

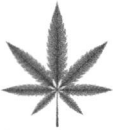

These symptoms can include irritability, anxiety, mood changes, sleep disturbances, decreased appetite, and cravings for cannabis. However, the severity and duration of these symptoms can vary widely among individuals.

164

Some Social Challenges and Complications of Cannabis Use

The complexity of cannabis as a plant and the variability in its active ingredients can pose legal and medical challenges. Here're some of the critical issues:

- **Legal Implications**: The varying legal status of cannabis in different jurisdictions complicates the situation. In some places, cannabis may be permitted for recreational or medicinal use, while in others, it remains illegal for any purpose. This creates challenges in terms of regulation, drug testing, and establishing legal limits for impairment, especially when it comes to driving under the influence.
- **Standardized Testing**: Determining the rate

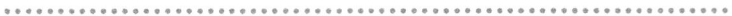

of elimination of cannabis from your body can be challenging due to the presence of multiple active compounds and variations in individual metabolism.

While cannabis can be detected in urine, blood, saliva, and hair tests, interpreting these results can be complex.

The presence of cannabis metabolites in these tests doesn't necessarily indicate recent use or impairment, as they can persist in the body for an extended period after use.

- **Medical Treatment**: The interactions between cannabis and other drugs, including prescription medications, can be a concern. Cannabis use may affect the metabolism and efficacy of other medications, potentially leading to unpredictable drug interactions and therapeutic outcomes. This highlights the importance of healthcare professionals being aware of a patient's cannabis use and considering it when prescribing medications.
- **Individual Variations:** People can have different responses to cannabis due to variations in metabolism, enzyme activity, and other individual factors.

  This can make establishing standardized guidelines for dosing, monitoring, and treatment challenging.
- **Research and Education**: Due to the legal and regulatory restrictions surrounding cannabis, research on its effects, interactions, and long-term consequences is still evolving. More research is needed to better understand the potential risks, benefits, and interactions associated with cannabis use.

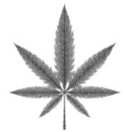

165

It's crucial for policymakers, healthcare professionals, and individuals to stay informed about the legal and medical implications of cannabis use and to promote

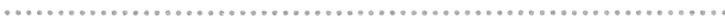

evidence-based approaches to address the associated challenges.

Cannabis Use and Legal Challenges

The legal implications of someone acting intoxicated due to the release of cannabis from their storage sites can be complex and may vary depending on the jurisdiction. Here are some points to consider:

- **Impairment and Legal Responsibility**: If a person is exhibiting signs of intoxication or impairment due to the release of cannabis from their fatty tissues, it can raise questions about their legal responsibility for their actions. In legal systems that consider impairment as a basis for liability, it may be challenging to determine whether the person's behaviour was influenced by recent cannabis use or the release of stored cannabis. This could potentially impact their legal responsibility for any actions taken during that time.
- **Drug Testing and Interpretation**: Blood tests may detect the presence of cannabis or its metabolites, but the timing of use can be difficult to establish accurately. While blood tests can show the same levels of cannabis as if it was ingested recently, it may not necessarily reflect recent use, especially if cannabis is being released from fatty tissues. In such cases, additional evidence and expert testimony may be required to provide a more comprehensive understanding of the situation.
- **Defences and Mitigating Factors**: In legal proceedings, the individual may raise defences or present mitigating factors to argue that their actions were involuntary

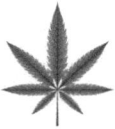

or influenced by factors beyond their control. This could include presenting evidence of the release of stored cannabis or other physiological effects that contributed to their behaviour. The acceptance and viability of such defences can vary depending on the specific legal jurisdiction and the circumstances of the case.

It's important to consult legal professionals familiar with the laws and regulations in your jurisdiction to obtain accurate and up-to-date information regarding the legal implications of cannabis use. Laws and interpretations can differ, and legal advice should be sought from qualified professionals.

Cannabis, Impairment and Accidents

In determining legal responsibility in cases involving drug impairment and accidents, legal implications can vary depending on the specific circumstances and the jurisdiction in which the incident occurred. Here are some general considerations:

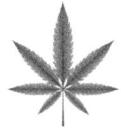

167

- **Impairment and Traffic Laws**: If a driver is impaired by any substance, whether legal or illegal, it can lead to legal consequences if it's determined to be a contributing factor to an accident. Traffic laws typically prohibit driving under the influence of drugs or alcohol, and violations of these laws can result in penalties.
- **Legal Limits and Prescription Drugs**: In the case of legal substances such as alcohol or prescription drugs, jurisdictions often define legal limits or provide guidelines for safe usage. If a driver exceeds the legal limits or operates a vehicle while impaired by prescription medication without a valid prescription or against medical advice, they may face legal repercussions.

- **Doctor-Patient Responsibility**: In situations involving prescription drugs, the responsibility of doctors to inform patients about potential impairing effects can come into question. Suppose a doctor fails to provide adequate warnings or instructions regarding the potential impact of a prescribed medication on a patient's ability to operate machinery or drive safely. In that case, the prescribing doctor may be held accountable for any resulting harm.
- **Illegal Drugs**: If a driver was impaired by an illegal drug at the time of an accident, it could lead to criminal charges. Possession or use of illegal drugs can carry legal penalties. If their impairment is determined to have caused the accident, the legal consequences can be severe, including jail time.

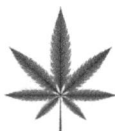

Cannabis, Pregnancy, and the Law

168

Cannabis, with its unpredictable effects, poses interesting challenges when it comes to the law. Let's start with pregnant women, shall we? Now, we know that cannabis can pass through the placenta, making its way to the developing baby. As pregnancy progresses, women tend to gain weight, which unfortunately means they also accumulate more cannabis in their bodies.

When it comes to the legal implications, things get even more intriguing. While cannabis may be permitted in certain jurisdictions, the use of cannabis during pregnancy is often a gray area. There're still many unanswered questions about how cannabis affects the developing fetus and the long-term consequences it may have. Researchers are working hard to understand these effects, but we're left with a lot of uncertainty for now.

If a pregnant woman uses cannabis for nausea, morn-

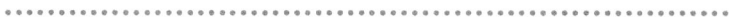

ing sickness, anxiety, or pain, and something goes awry, legal complications arise. Was the woman aware of the potential risks of cannabis use during pregnancy? Did her healthcare provider adequately inform her about the potential dangers? It's like a game of "who knew what when." If the healthcare provider failed to provide proper guidance, they might be in hot water.

It's well-known that cannabis use can negatively impact brain development, particularly in individuals under twenty-five. The developing brain is highly vulnerable to the effects of substances like cannabis, and this vulnerability extends to the **prenatal period**.

When a pregnant woman uses cannabis, the drug can cross the placenta and reach the developing baby. This means that the unborn child's developing brain may be exposed to cannabis and its active components.

169

Research suggests that exposure to cannabis during pregnancy may disrupt normal brain development in the fetus. The endocannabinoid system, which plays a crucial role in brain development, can be influenced by the active compounds in cannabis. This interference can potentially lead to long-term consequences for the child's cognitive function, learning abilities, and emotional well-being.

It's important to note that the specific effects of prenatal cannabis exposure are still being actively studied, and more research is needed to fully understand the extent of the risks involved. However, based on current knowledge about the effects of cannabis on the developing brain, pregnant women should avoid cannabis use to minimize any potential harm to their unborn.

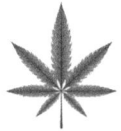

A circus clown was entertaining a crowd by doing "clown stuff," non-verbal goofing to make people laugh. He performed a couple of impressive tricks that wowed the crowd, especially his juggling skills.

He then performed another juggling trick that caused some to be concerned right off the bet. He was going to juggle marbles with his mouth. The clown knew some people were skeptical about his trick, so he played with their minds a little more.

He would toss the marbles a few times and then pretend that he had swallowed one of them. He took the trick further. He juggled the marbles and then made it appear as though the marble had tumbled down the wrong pipe, and he was choking.

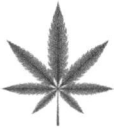

People would run to try and help him, but only to realize he was playing with them. He did that a couple of times, and then people stopped rushing to him each time he pretended to choke—they'd just watch and laugh.

Unbeknownst to him, fate had other plans for him as he attempted the trick one last time, and this time the marble really fell down the wrong pipe. As he tried to signal for help, the crowd laughed, especially at how convincing his cry for help had become.

The makeup made seeing his skin turning blue nearly impossible as he was suffocating. He didn't make it, but at least he died doing what he loved.

Some Makeup For The Doctor?

Getting medical help

The most common reasons for visiting a physician range from reproductive issues–missed periods and **erectile dysfunction**–to pain and general discomfort. A patient can present to the doctor complaining about worsening fatigue. An examination and some tests may reveal that the patient has cancer or another debilitating condition. Most patients with vague symptoms such as fatigue, loss of appetite, excessive sleeping, and so on go to their doctors hoping to get answers.

Some people increasingly consult "Dr. Google" first, then head to the doctor to request a specific prescription. The goal of a doctor is to educate you so you understand what's going on with your health. While educating yourself and being informed can be beneficial, it's crucial to approach online information cautiously, as it may not always be accurate or applicable to individual cases. This'll enable you to understand how to best manage your circumstances.

171

Visiting a doctor allows for a comprehensive evaluation of symptoms, medical history, and physical examination, which are crucial for proper diagnosis and management. Doctors have the expertise to interpret the complex interplay of symptoms and guide patients toward appropriate treatment options or further investigations if needed. They aim to educate patients about their health conditions, giving them a deeper understanding of the underlying issues and empowering them to participate in their healthcare actively.

It's essential for patients to actively engage in discussions with their doctors, asking questions and expressing concerns. This collaborative approach ensures that patients are well-informed and can make informed decisions about their health management, considering their unique circumstances and preferences.

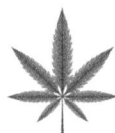

Understanding Therapeutic alliance

Yes, we've developed a considerable lag in the trust between doctors and patients, leading to more and more people resorting to self-medicating with unconventional and questionable methods. It's neither the doctors' nor the patients' fault. The overabundance and easy accessibility of information based on **anecdotal evidence** but presented as facts is one of the culprits to blame. This can lead to patients seeking unconventional or questionable methods of self-medication. For example, "I took this herb for my abdominal pain that wasn't going away with over-the-counter pain medication. It's been months since I felt any kind of abdominal pain. You should try this herb too for your pain or that other discomfort that bothers you a lot."

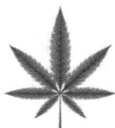

It's essential to recognize that building a sustainable healthcare system relies on collaboration between knowledgeable medical professionals and compliant, open-minded patients. This collaboration forms what's known as a **therapeutic alliance**—a relationship based on mutual trust, respect, and shared goals.

In a therapeutic alliance, doctors and patients work together as a team, with the doctor providing expertise, guidance, and evidence-based information. In contrast, the patient actively participates in decision-making and follows the recommended treatment plans. Open and honest communication is critical to establishing this alliance, allowing patients to express their concerns, ask questions, and seek clarification about their health conditions and treatment options.

When patients encounter anecdotal evidence or alternative approaches, doctors must provide clear explanations backed by scientific evidence to help them make informed health decisions. Doctors can educate patients about different interventions' potential risks and benefits, including conventional treatments and complementary or alternative therapies.

Ethical regulators, such as medical boards and professional associations, ensure that healthcare providers uphold standards of practice and ethical conduct. They help maintain the integrity of the healthcare system by promoting evidence-based medicine, patient safety, and professional accountability.

We can strengthen the healthcare system and improve patient outcomes by fostering a strong therapeutic alliance where doctors and patients work collaboratively and trust each other's efforts to achieve positive patient outcomes.

The Rise of Alternative Medicine

When faced with severe pain or discomfort, it's understandable that some patients may be willing to explore alternative medicine or unconventional treatments in search of relief. The desire to find relief is a natural response to suffering, and individuals may be motivated by a sense of desperation.

173

Alternative medicine refers to medical practices not part of conventional Western medicine and may not have a scientific basis. While some alternative therapies may provide comfort or a placebo effect, their effectiveness in treating specific health conditions often needs to be proven or supported by rigorous scientific research. This can include practices like Acupuncture, Chiropractic, Herbal medicine, Homeopathy, Massage therapy, Yoga, Reiki, Aromatherapy, Tai chi, Naturopathy, Ayurveda, and Mind-body therapies like meditation and hypnotherapy.
Healthcare professionals, including doctors, are responsible for educating patients about the potential risks and benefits of alternative therapies. They should

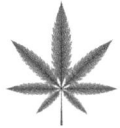

provide evidence-based information and guide patients toward treatments that have been scientifically validated and proven to be safe and effective. Doctors need to stay up-to-date with medical knowledge and continue their professional development to provide the best care for their patients.

Health regulators are crucial in ensuring ethical practices and protecting patient welfare. However, as with any profession, there's always the potential for unethical behaviour or self-interest. Vigilance and accountability are necessary to ensure that health regulators uphold the highest standards of ethics and prioritize patient well-being.

Ultimately, patients have the right to make decisions about their healthcare, including exploring alternative options. However, they must be aware of the potential limitations, risks, and lack of scientific evidence associated with alternative medicine. Open communication between patients and healthcare providers can help patients make informed choices and understand the potential consequences of their decisions.

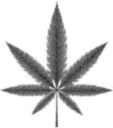

174

The Questionable Practice of Self-medication

Treating symptoms without addressing the underlying cause of the symptoms can be compared to using duct tape to fix a cracked wall in your house. While it may provide temporary relief, it doesn't address the root issue, which may persist or worsen over time.

When patients take it upon themselves to self-treat their symptoms, there're potential risks and limitations to consider. Individuals may misdiagnose their condition without proper medical training and knowledge or overlook more serious underlying causes. This can lead to delayed or inadequate treatment and potentially worsening of the disease.
Furthermore, self-treatment may involve using over-the-counter medications or alternative therapies that may not be appropriate or effective for

the specific condition. There's also the risk of drug interactions or adverse effects if self-medication isn't done correctly or without proper guidance from a healthcare professional.

While self-care practices, such as rest, staying hydrated, and managing minor symptoms, can be helpful in certain situations, it's essential to know when to seek professional medical advice. Medical professionals have the expertise and diagnostic tools to accurately assess your condition, identify underlying causes, and provide appropriate treatment.

A collaborative approach between patients and healthcare professionals is crucial for effective and safe healthcare. Patients should communicate their symptoms, concerns, and any self-treatments they have tried to their healthcare provider. This allows the healthcare provider to make a comprehensive assessment, provide an accurate diagnosis, and recommend appropriate treatment options based on your specific needs.

175

Relying solely on anecdotal experiences and seeking advice from friends or acquaintances can be a common practice for some individuals when it comes to managing their health. While sharing personal experiences and seeking support from others can be beneficial in certain situations, it's essential to recognize this approach's limitations and potential risks.

Self-diagnosis: Playing with Fire

Fake doctors—quarks—treat symptoms, good doctors treat diseases, and great doctors treat patients. Treating symptoms is like fixing a cracked wall with duct tape; only quarks fix health problems like that. The problem is that while you can take a pill to alleviate a fever, an infection that could be causing the fever—which needs an antibiotic to be treated—might be getting worse. On the other hand, if you find out

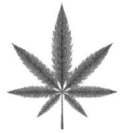

what caused the fever and address that instead, you may do a better job in less time while producing the most effective results.

Each person's health condition and medical history are unique, and what works for one individual may not work for another. Symptoms can vary significantly in terms of severity, underlying causes, and appropriate treatment options. Relying solely on the experiences and advice of others may lead to misdiagnosis or ineffective treatments, as different conditions may require specific medical interventions or therapies.

Medical professionals undergo years of training and education to develop the expertise necessary to diagnose and treat various health conditions accurately. They have access to evidence-based guidelines, medical research, diagnostic tools, and a comprehensive understanding of the complexities of the human body. Consulting with a healthcare professional provides the opportunity for a thorough evaluation, proper diagnosis, and personalized treatment plan based on your specific needs.

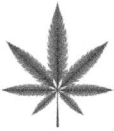

176

While it's understandable that some individuals may feel reluctant to seek medical care, it's essential to prioritize your health and make informed decisions. Healthcare professionals are there to provide knowledge, guidance, support, and appropriate medical interventions to ensure the best possible outcomes for patients.

Some people have lived for years without seeing a family physician. They rely on finding out who in their circles has experienced similar symptoms. They then ask what the friend did to treat those symptoms, and they'll do the same to treat their own symptoms.

It's the story about Man A, who developed symptoms 1 and 2, and he decided to ask Man B if Man B ever developed symptoms 1 and 2. If Man B admits to having once developed symptoms 1 and 2, Man A will inquire what Man B did to get rid of symptoms 1 and 2. If Man B successfully got rid of symptoms 1 and 2, Man A will do precisely what he's told by Man B. If Man B failed to eliminate symptoms 1 and 2, Man A will move on to Man C, D, E, etc. Only when there's nowhere else to look will Man A turn to a physician.

This's the same story, with some men refusing to ask for directions. When they finally admit to themselves that they're lost, they'll secretly turn on the GPS and plug in their concealed earpiece. Some call it taking charge, but this's just plain ignorance gone wild.

Patient Education and Empowerment

It's crucial for patients to have access to accurate and reliable information about their health, conditions, and treatment options. Understandably, patients may sometimes feel frustrated with the healthcare system. However, it's important to remember that medical professionals undergo extensive training to acquire the necessary knowledge and skills to provide appropriate care. Self-diagnosis and self-treatment can be risky because individuals may not have the same expertise or access to comprehensive medical resources.

177

The risks of self-diagnosis and self-treatment include:

- Misdiagnosis.
- Delayed or inadequate treatment.
- Worsening of symptoms or underlying conditions.
- Potential drug interactions or adverse reactions.

Additionally, some health conditions may have overlapping symptoms, making it challenging for individuals without medical training to identify the underlying cause accurately.

Promoting patient education and health literacy is crucial to empower individuals to make informed decisions about their health. This can be achieved through initiatives that provide accessible and reliable health information, encourage open communication between patients and healthcare professionals, and promote shared decision-making in treatment plans.

By fostering a collaborative relationship between patients and healthcare providers, patients can better understand their conditions, treatment options, potential risks, and benefits. This can help patients make more informed choices and actively participate in their healthcare. It's important to emphasize that while patient education is crucial, it should complement and not replace professional medical care.

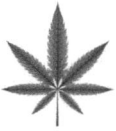

In all fairness, our healthcare system has failed patients, and these patients have every right to take matters into their own hands. Is it safe, though? As a desperate means to an end, it doesn't matter to patients in most cases. The problem isn't resources; it's not knowing the risks and complications of "playing doctor" on themselves or their friends and family.

178

Short-term Benefits with Long-term Consequences
In the sixties, a drug was developed to treat morning sickness in pregnant women. This drug worked wonders, and women were happy with the drug until decades later. This drug was linked to cancer in daughters born to women who used that drug while pregnant. This drug was taken off the market.

We have talked about treating symptoms and leaving the underlying disease raging on. Now we see that the disease may have been cured, but future generations may suffer the adverse effects of the drug.
This incident underscores the importance of thorough research, rigorous testing, and ongoing monitoring of medications and treatments. While drugs may initially appear effective in relieving symptoms or addressing

specific conditions, their long-term effects may not always be fully understood or anticipated.

The field of medicine continually evolves as new information and evidence emerge. As we gain more knowledge about the complexities of diseases, genetics, and the effects of medications, it becomes essential to reassess treatments and make necessary adjustments to ensure patient safety.

In instances where potential risks or adverse effects are identified, regulatory bodies and healthcare providers should take action to mitigate harm. This can involve measures such as recalling drugs, updating prescribing guidelines, providing patient warnings and information, and conducting further research to understand the implications better.

The Misguided Confidence in Cannabis' Therapeutic Use

Cannabis has been used for various purposes, including alleviating symptoms associated with pain, depression, and morning sickness. However, it's essential to note that cannabis hasn't been proven to cure or treat specific diseases like some pharmaceuticals have been validated through rigorous clinical trials.

179

When a patient seeks medical care, a doctor's evaluation aims to identify the underlying problem or disease. Based on this assessment, a treatment plan is developed, which may involve addressing the root cause as well as providing symptomatic relief. **Symptomatic relief** focuses on managing and reducing the symptoms associated with a particular condition without necessarily targeting the underlying cause. Symptomatic relief aims to improve the patient's quality of life by reducing pain, discomfort, or other unpleasant symptoms.
Pharmaceutical medications can also involve symptomatic relief, where the goal is to improve the patient's quality of life by alleviating pain, discomfort, or

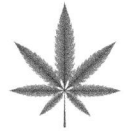

other distressing symptoms. These medications are often developed and tested through rigorous scientific research and clinical trials to ensure their safety and effectiveness.

While managing pain and discomfort can provide temporary relief, it's crucial to understand the cause of these symptoms to prevent further complications or worsening of the underlying condition.

When individuals experience persistent pain or discomfort, seeking medical attention allows for a thorough evaluation and diagnosis. Medical professionals can conduct tests, such as imaging studies or laboratory tests, to identify the underlying cause of the symptoms. This diagnostic process helps determine the appropriate course of treatment, which may involve addressing the root cause of the problem in addition to managing the symptoms.

For example, in the case of a fractured bone, relying solely on pain relief medications without proper medical intervention and stabilization may lead to further damage, delayed healing, or improper alignment of the bone. In the case of an ulcer, symptomatic relief alone may not address the underlying cause, such as an infection or an underlying condition like H. pylori infection. Delaying appropriate treatment of the ulcer can result in complications such as **perforation** or bleeding.

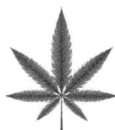

Imagine how many women might have used cannabis in the past for their morning sickness during pregnancy. Since cannabis passes through the placenta to dissolve in the tissues of the unborn child, a drug that benefits expectant mothers would likely harm that child irreparably. The prevalence of Autism Spectrum Disorders is at an all-time high, and any possible causes should be investigated.

This's not to say that only cannabis causes this impairment of brain function. Instead, all drugs that cross the placenta and can affect the brain in any way should also be studied. With the rise in the use of antidepressants, opioids, cannabis, and other re-

180

lated drugs, and the concurrent rise in **autism spectrum disorders**, we may end up normalizing what should be considered unethical. Studies have shown that exposure to cannabis during pregnancy may adversely affect fetal development, including potential impacts on brain development. However, it's essential to note that the research in this area is still evolving, and more studies are needed to establish a clear cause-and-effect relationship.

Autism spectrum disorders (ASD) encompass a range of neurodevelopmental conditions that affect individuals differently. While the exact cause of ASD is still not fully understood, research suggests a combination of genetic and environmental factors contribute to its development.
ASD can manifest in various ways and may present differently in each individual. Some individuals with ASD may have significant challenges with communication, while others may have relatively good language skills but struggle with social interactions. Restricted and repetitive patterns of behaviour, interests, or activities are also commonly observed in individuals with ASD.

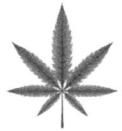

181

It's important to note that autism is a lifelong condition, and early intervention and support can significantly improve outcomes for individuals with ASD. Treatment approaches often involve a multidisciplinary approach, including behavioural therapies, educational support, speech therapy, and other interventions tailored to the individual's specific needs.
A person may experience severe headaches, dizziness, or morning sickness. These all seem like benign symptoms, but further investigation by a medical professional may reveal something as serious as a brain tumour. Suppose someone takes a drug like cannabis to self-medicate and suppress those symptoms for months or even years. In that case, the underlying tumour could continue growing wild, unchecked. It's crucial to understand that symptoms are the body's way of signalling that something is wrong, and sup-

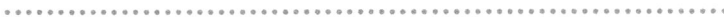

pressing those symptoms without proper medical evaluation can delay the diagnosis and appropriate treatment of an underlying condition.

While some symptoms may seem benign or easily manageable, they can sometimes indicate more serious underlying health issues, such as a brain tumour. Brain tumours, for instance, can initially present with symptoms like headaches or dizziness, which may be mistakenly attributed to other causes or temporarily relieved by self-medication. However, delaying medical evaluation can allow the tumour to progress unchecked, potentially leading to more severe complications and a poorer prognosis. Once more severe symptoms like unexplained weight loss are noticed, the patient might consult a physician. The problem is that it may be too late.

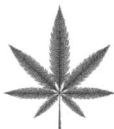

Most diseases present as **non-specific symptoms** like fever, dizziness, fatigue, cough, pain, etc. All of these symptoms can be treated with cannabis, but the danger is that they're only symptoms, and the underlying disease remains unnoticed. Symptoms may be relieved for some time, but the disease will show up sooner or later.

A prevalent example is erectile dysfunction in men over the age of fifty. It's now a common medical principle that any man over the age of fifty with erectile dysfunction should be tested for **diabetes mellitus**. One of the underlying causes of erectile dysfunction in men with diabetes mellitus is the damage to blood vessels and nerves of their genitals that can occur due to chronically elevated blood sugar levels. However, most men over fifty will first seek help from "the blue pill." While the blue pill gets the equipment up and running, the possibility of high blood sugar will remain unchecked. This increased blood sugar can lead to limp amputations, kidney disease, stroke, blindness, fatal heart disease, and even coma.

This's not a theory, but something already happening in our society.

Various factors, including cardiac issues like blocked coronary arteries, can cause chest pain. While strong painkillers may provide temporary relief from chest pain, it is crucial to understand the underlying cause of the pain. Ignoring or dismissing chest pain without proper evaluation can be risky, as it may delay the diagnosis and appropriate management of potentially serious conditions.

Heart disease, including conditions like coronary artery disease, can lead to the development of blockages in the blood vessels that supply the heart. These blockages can restrict blood flow to the heart muscle, leading to chest pain or discomfort, known as angina. If left untreated, these blockages can eventually lead to a heart attack, which can be life-threatening.
When discussing masking diseases by treating symptoms, the word "long" is highly subjective. "Long" could be years for cancer or minutes for a heart attack. Either way, you can't afford to take your chances by focusing only on the symptoms. Instead, spend time finding someone who can explain why the symptoms are there in the first place.

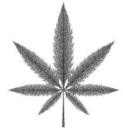

183

Ms. X was visiting a small village in Africa. She saw women leaving their homes after breakfast to fetch water, only to return home in time for dinner. She was disheartened and vowed to do something to end the problem these women were facing.

Ms. X travelled back to her country and returned with enough resources to build a borehole in this small village. This new source of clean water was close enough to the entire village to cut the time needed to fetch water from ten hours to less than one hour. Ms. X left the village and the country happy that she had made a significant, positive difference.

Ms. X returned to the African village after a few months to check on her helpful deed and see if she could do more. She was shocked to see the borehole broken and non-functional. She couldn't understand why people wouldn't care for something meant to solve their problems.

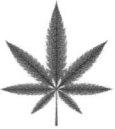

184

After consulting with other women in that small village, she discovered that the men were the problem. These men were so irritating that the only way for wives to get some peace was to be away for the entire day. When the borehole was built, it meant women would spend more time with their irritating husbands. The women found a simple solution to the problem: they broke the borehole.

When The Best Turns Out To Be The Worst

The Evil Drug That's Also Amazing

The discussion surrounding cannabis has been complex and influenced by various factors, including social perceptions and individual experiences. While cannabis has been used for medicinal purposes and has shown potential benefits in managing specific conditions, it's crucial to approach its use with caution and a scientific perspective.

THC and CBD interact with specific receptors in your body's endocannabinoid system. This interaction can result in various effects, including pain relief, mood alteration, and appetite stimulation. Of course, watching your mother in pain is unbearable. However, watching your mother with the munchies trying to engage in a fistfight with a mosquito can bring a different kind of pain.

185

In the context of medical use, cannabis has demonstrated effectiveness in alleviating pain, reducing nausea and vomiting in cancer patients undergoing chemotherapy, and improving appetite in individuals with conditions like HIV/AIDS. It may also have potential therapeutic effects on certain mental health disorders, such as reducing anxiety or aiding sleep.

However, it's crucial to recognize that cannabis isn't without risks. The psychoactive effects of THC can lead to cognitive impairment, memory problems, and increased heart rate. Prolonged or heavy cannabis use, particularly in susceptible individuals, may also increase the risk of developing mental health issues, including psychosis or worsening symptoms in individuals already predisposed to psychiatric conditions. Based on current knowl-

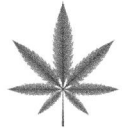

edge, cannabis can help with mental health problems and also cause mental health problems.

To ensure the responsible use of cannabis for medical purposes, further research is needed to better understand its potential benefits, risks, and optimal dosages for specific conditions. This includes investigating different strains, formulations, and delivery methods to maximize therapeutic effects while minimizing unwanted side effects.

Moreover, it's crucial to approach cannabis use within a framework of harm reduction. This means promoting safe and informed use, educating on potential risks, and encouraging individuals to consult healthcare professionals for guidance, particularly when managing complex medical conditions or mental health concerns.

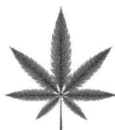

186

By continuing scientific research, fostering open dialogue, and implementing evidence-based regulations, we can strive to strike a balance between harnessing the potential benefits of cannabis for medical use and minimizing potential harm.

Science: A Systematic Approach to the World

Science is a structured approach that allows us to observe and understand the natural world carefully and systematically. Through scientific investigation, we aim to gather reliable evidence and knowledge that can be replicated and tested under various conditions. For something to be considered a scientific fact, it must be objectively observed and have practical applications beyond a single situation.

When it comes to harm reduction, applying a scientific approach can benefit people worldwide. By objectively examining the evidence and considering a range of settings and circumstances, we can develop strategies and interventions that minimize harm and maximize benefits.

When implementing harm reduction strategies, it's vital to distinguish between subjective experiences and objective observations. Personal perspectives, biases, and individual circumstances influence subjective experiences. At the same time, objective observations are based on systematic data collection and analysis. Relying solely on subjective experiences can lead to biased recommendations that may have different outcomes in different settings.

To ensure effective harm reduction, scientific studies and research are crucial. These studies help us gather reliable evidence and evaluate the impact of interventions in different populations and contexts. By conducting rigorous experiments, analyzing data, and seeking peer review, scientists can provide accurate and well-informed recommendations for harm reduction practices.

187

By embracing a scientific approach to harm reduction, we can enhance our understanding of the risks and benefits associated with various behaviours, substances, or practices. This knowledge can guide the development of evidence-based strategies that prioritize safety and promote the well-being of individuals and communities.

Understanding Harm Reduction

Methadone clinics play a crucial role in the treatment of opioid addiction. **Methadone**, a medication used in medication-assisted treatment, helps individuals struggling with **opioid addiction** by relieving cravings and withdrawal symptoms. This allows patients to stabilize their lives and engage in the recovery process.

The use of methadone in opioid addiction treatment follows a two-step process. Initially, methadone is

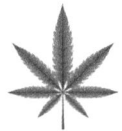

substituted for the opioids on which the individual depends. This substitution helps reduce withdrawal symptoms and cravings, enabling the patient to function without the harmful effects of illicit opioid use. The second step involves gradually tapering off the dose of methadone, with the ultimate goal of achieving abstinence from all opioids.

Methadone clinics adhere to a standardized approach that prioritizes the safety and well-being of patients. The clinics provide comprehensive care, including regular medical check-ups, counselling, and support services, to address the physical, psychological, and social aspects of addiction recovery.

It's important to note that the effectiveness of methadone treatment can vary among individuals. Factors such as the severity of addiction, individual response to medication, and the presence of co-occurring mental health conditions can influence treatment outcomes. Additionally, medication-assisted treatment with methadone is often accompanied by behavioural therapies and support programs to enhance the chances of long-term recovery.

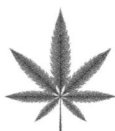

While methadone treatment has been widely adopted and proven beneficial for many individuals, it's essential to continue research and evaluation to improve its effectiveness and address any potential limitations. Ongoing studies and advancements in addiction medicine aim to enhance treatment options and develop personalized approaches tailored to each patient's needs.

Differences in Harm Reduction

Approaches to addressing the opioid crisis differ between regions, such as North America and certain European countries. Societal values, cultural perspectives, and differing interpretations of scientific evidence can influence these variations. While it's essential to consider various approaches, it's crucial to base interventions on scientific merits and evidence-based practices to ensure the best outcomes.

In North America, efforts to combat the opioid crisis have involved a range of strategies, including harm reduction approaches such as providing clean needles and opioid replacement therapies like methadone. These approaches aim to reduce the harms associated with opioid use, such as the spread of infectious diseases and overdose deaths. Harm reduction recognizes the reality that some individuals may continue to use drugs and seeks to minimize the associated risks.

On the other hand, in certain European countries, there has been a stronger emphasis on abstinence-based treatment approaches, which prioritize helping individuals overcome addiction without using opioids or other substitute medications. These approaches focus on comprehensive treatment, rehabilitation, and support services to promote long-term recovery.

189

It's important to note that the opioid crisis is a complex issue with multiple underlying factors, including the overprescribing of opioids, socioeconomic factors, and the presence of illicit drug markets. Finding practical solutions requires a comprehensive understanding of these underlying problems and addressing them in a multifaceted manner.

While harm reduction strategies have shown some positive outcomes in terms of reducing certain harms associated with drug use, such as HIV transmission and overdose deaths, they aren't without limitations. It's essential to continuously evaluate and adapt interventions based on scientific evidence and the evolving understanding of addiction treatment.

Efforts to combat the opioid crisis should incorporate a range of approaches, including prevention, treatment, and harm reduction strategies, while also

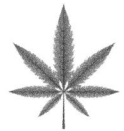

considering the individual needs and circumstances of those affected by opioid addiction. Collaborative efforts between healthcare professionals, policymakers, and communities are necessary to develop comprehensive and practical solutions.

When Money Speaks Louder

The pharmaceutical industry and the regulation of drugs can be complex and influenced by various factors, including economic considerations. It's essential to ensure that the healthcare system prioritizes the well-being of individuals and public health over financial gains.

While certain drugs, such as alcohol and tobacco, have been linked to significant health problems, they remain legal and widely available in many countries. These substances pose substantial health risks, leading to diseases and premature deaths. The reasons for their continued legality and commercial success can be attributed to various factors, including historical and cultural acceptance, tax revenue, industry lobbying, and economic considerations.

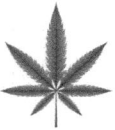

190

Addressing the harmful effects of drugs like alcohol and tobacco requires a comprehensive approach that includes public health campaigns, regulations, and support for prevention and treatment programs. Governments and regulatory bodies must prioritize public health and make evidence-based decisions regarding drug regulation and policies.

Promoting ethical practices and responsible decision-making within the pharmaceutical industry and healthcare system is crucial to protect the well-being of individuals and prevent the collapse of the healthcare system. Transparency, rigorous evaluation of drug safety and efficacy, and the consideration of long-term health consequences should be integral parts of the drug regulatory process.

Efforts should also address the social determinants of drug abuse and addiction, including poverty, inequality, and access to healthcare and social support systems. Collaborative efforts involving policymakers, healthcare professionals, public health experts, and communities are necessary to advocate for ethical practices, improve drug regulation, and promote the well-being of individuals and society as a whole.

Tobacco: A Cautionary Tale

The history of tobacco serves as a cautionary tale highlighting the importance of transparency, accurate information, and responsible drug regulation. The case of tobacco is a significant example of a product marketed and sold for recreational use without fully understanding its addictive nature and long-term health consequences.

Tobacco was promoted as a stress-relieving and enjoyable product when it was first introduced. However, the addictive nature of nicotine, the main psychoactive component of tobacco, was not fully disclosed or widely known at the time. As years went by, the detrimental health effects of tobacco use became increasingly evident, with a strong association between smoking and various types of cancer, heart disease, and other serious health conditions.

191

The tobacco industry has faced numerous lawsuits and paid substantial amounts in punitive damages due to the harmful effects of its products. These legal actions have brought attention to the deceptive marketing practices employed by tobacco companies and the devastating impact of tobacco use on public health.

The lessons learned from the tobacco industry can certainly inform discussions about other substances, including cannabis. It's crucial to approach the legalization and regulation of cannabis with a strong em-

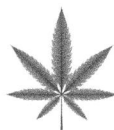

phasis on scientific research, public health considerations, and informed decision-making. Transparency
about the potential risks and benefits of cannabis,
including its addictive potential, is essential in providing individuals with accurate information to make informed choices about their health.

As cannabis use becomes more widespread and its
potential therapeutic applications are explored, it's
vital to prioritize rigorous scientific research, comprehensive education campaigns, and responsible regulation. By learning from past experiences, society can
aim to strike a balance between the potential benefits
of cannabis and the need to mitigate potential risks
and ensure public safety.

Trusting a Doctor's Recommendations

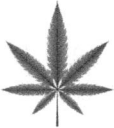

Establishing a strong and trusting relationship between doctors and patients is crucial for effective
healthcare delivery. This relationship is often referred to as the therapeutic alliance, built on the understanding that the doctor possesses expertise and
knowledge in medicine, and the patient seeks their
guidance and care.

192

In the ideal scenario, patients rely on doctors to provide accurate information, educate them about their
health conditions, and offer appropriate treatment
options. On the other hand, doctors devote their time,
skills, and knowledge to diagnosing and treating patients, aiming for positive health outcomes.
However, trust can be undermined in various ways.
One significant issue is when doctors fail to stay updated with the latest medical knowledge or rely on unreliable sources of information. Patients expect their
doctors to have access to credible resources and up-
to-date research to provide accurate diagnoses and
evidence-based treatment recommendations. Suppose patients perceive that their doctor lacks knowledge or is using unreliable sources. In that case, it can

erode their trust in the doctor's competence and the advice they provide.

Conversely, patients who disregard their doctor's recommendations or fail to engage in their own healthcare actively can also strain the therapeutic alliance. Healthcare is a collaborative effort, and patients are responsible for actively participating in their own care by following medical advice, adhering to treatment plans, and maintaining open communication with their doctors. When patients consistently ignore or dismiss medical advice, it can be disheartening for doctors and hinder the effectiveness of the treatment.

Doctors must prioritize continuous education and stay updated with the latest research and medical advancements to foster trust and strengthen the therapeutic alliance. Open and honest communication between doctors and patients, emphasizing shared decision-making, can also contribute to a more trusting relationship. Patients should feel comfortable asking questions and expressing their concerns, while doctors should actively listen and address their patients' needs.

193

Building a robust therapeutic alliance requires effort and commitment from both doctors and patients. Trust is earned through mutual respect, effective communication, and a shared commitment to achieving optimal health outcomes.

When a patient consistently fails to follow medical advice or make progress toward their health goals, it can strain the trust between the doctor and the patient.

In the case of weight loss, it's essential to recognize that changing habits and achieving sustainable weight management is a complex process that requires commitment and dedication from both the doctor and the patient. Doctors can provide guidance, support, and evidence-based strategies. At the same time,

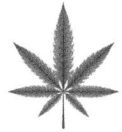

patients must actively engage in their health and make lifestyle changes.

When a patient repeatedly fails to follow through with the advice and does not make progress, it can be frustrating for both the doctor and the patient. It may lead to a sense of disappointment, and the doctor may feel less motivated to invest significant time and attention into a patient who doesn't seem receptive to their recommendations. This could strain the doctor-patient relationship and compromise the effectiveness of the healthcare provided.

To address this challenge, fostering open and honest communication between the doctor and the patient is crucial. Patients should feel comfortable expressing their struggles, challenges, and barriers to adherence. Doctors, in turn, should actively listen, understand, and provide support tailored to the individual patient's needs and circumstances. By working together and maintaining ongoing dialogue, doctors and patients can collaboratively develop realistic goals, strategies, and timelines for weight management.

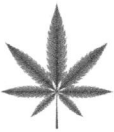

194

Additionally, it's crucial to recognize that weight management isn't solely the patient's responsibility. Healthcare systems should also focus on creating environments that support healthy lifestyles, provide resources for behaviour change, and address social determinants of health that may influence weight management outcomes.

By fostering a solid doctor-patient relationship based on trust, empathy, and shared decision-making, healthcare professionals can better support patients in their weight management journey. Ultimately, the collapse of the healthcare system can be mitigated by nurturing positive doctor-patient relationships and implementing comprehensive approaches to address the complexities of weight management.

The Power Struggle in Modern Healthcare

It's important to acknowledge that individuals can exhibit behaviours that aren't conducive to a positive doctor-patient relationship within any profession, including medicine. The notion of a "god complex" where a doctor asserts absolute authority and expects unquestioning obedience doesn't represent the ideal doctor-patient dynamic.

A healthy doctor-patient relationship should be mutual respect, open communication, and collaboration. Patients have the right to ask questions, seek clarification, and actively participate in their healthcare decisions. Doctors, in turn, should listen to their patients, address their concerns, and provide information to help them make informed choices.

Similarly, overutilizing healthcare resources can strain the system and contribute to inefficiencies. Some patients may seek medical attention for minor or non-urgent issues, which can divert resources and time from those who genuinely need immediate care. This's why education and awareness campaigns promoting the appropriate use of healthcare services are valuable in order to ensure that resources are allocated effectively.

195

However, it's vital to approach this issue with empathy and understanding. Patients may have different levels of health literacy, anxiety about their symptoms, or cultural beliefs that influence their healthcare-seeking behaviour. Rather than blaming patients, educating and empowering individuals to make informed decisions about their health is essential while promoting responsible use of healthcare resources.

Addressing these various challenges from all angles is necessary to strengthen the healthcare system. This includes fostering professionalism and empathy among healthcare providers, promoting patient education

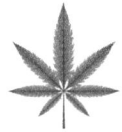

and empowerment, implementing evidence-based guidelines for appropriate healthcare utilization, and continuously improving access to healthcare services for all individuals.

The popularity of unconventional healing methods and the use of herbs and alternative drugs with unproven claims can be attributed to several factors. While medical doctors are scientists who rely on evidence-based practices, the appeal of unconventional methods often lies in their perceived naturalness, cultural traditions, and the desire for a more holistic approach to health and well-being.

It's essential to recognize that not all alternative therapies or herbal remedies have been extensively studied or subjected to rigorous scientific scrutiny. The lack of scientific evidence doesn't necessarily mean these methods are ineffective. Still, it does highlight the need for caution and critical evaluation.

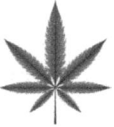

196

Sometimes, individuals may turn to alternative methods because they have had negative experiences with the conventional healthcare system, feel unheard, or seek more personalized and patient-centred care. They may also be drawn to taking an active role in their healing process and exploring a wide range of options.

However, it's crucial to approach these alternative methods with a critical mindset and seek reliable information and guidance from healthcare professionals. Integrative medicine, for example, combines evidence-based conventional medicine with complementary and alternative therapies in a coordinated and informed manner.

To address the challenges posed by the popularity of unproven alternative treatments, it's necessary to promote science literacy, critical thinking, and public awareness about evidence-based medicine. It's cru-

cial to create an environment of trust and open dialogue where patients feel comfortable discussing their healthcare choices and can make informed decisions.

The Scientific Approach with Data Analysis

It's essential to distinguish between valid scientific research and sensational claims that may lack scientific rigour or plausibility. While data analysis and statistical methods are vital tools in research, it's crucial to interpret the results meaningfully and scientifically soundly.

Correlation doesn't imply causation, and this principle is a fundamental aspect of scientific reasoning. Simply observing a correlation between two variables doesn't automatically mean that one variable causes the other. It's necessary to consider other factors, establish plausible mechanisms, and conduct rigorous studies to establish causality.

For example, think about someone claiming that toilet paper causes anal cancer because nearly everyone that has ever had anal cancer used toilet paper. This person will say that they can prove that claim with numbers. It doesn't take anything more than a minimally functional brain to realize that while the numbers do correlate, there's little to no association between anal cancer and the use of toilet paper. Someone else can claim that saliva can cause stomach cancer, especially if swallowed in small amounts over a long period. "Working backwards," they can further explain, "everyone with stomach cancer has a history of swallowing saliva in small amounts." That's everyone!

These claims rely on oversimplifying the data and disregarding critical contextual factors. Researchers are responsible for conducting rigorous studies, critically analyzing their findings, and presenting them in a balanced and evidence-based manner. The scientific community employs peer review processes to evaluate the quality and validity of research before it's published. However, it's important to note that there can

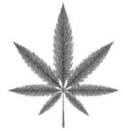

be differing opinions, ongoing debates, and revisions of conclusions based on new evidence, even in the scientific community.

To ensure the integrity and reliability of scientific research, scientists, journal editors, and the broader scientific community must uphold rigorous standards, engage in critical evaluation, and encourage transparency and reproducibility. It's also essential for the general public to be critical information consumers, seek reputable sources, and rely on a consensus of scientific evidence when making decisions about their health and well-being.

Establishing a cause-and-effect relationship in scientific research can be challenging. In many cases, researchers settle for identifying associations between variables. Association refers to the observed relationship between two variables, where changes in one variable are related to changes in another. This relationship can be identified through statistical analysis and observation of trends in the data.

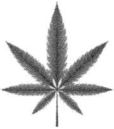

198

Associations can provide valuable insights and guide further investigation. They help researchers generate hypotheses and explore potential mechanisms underlying the observed relationship. However, it's essential to note that association doesn't imply causation. Identifying an association doesn't prove that one variable causes the other, as other factors or underlying mechanisms may be at play.

To establish causation, additional evidence is required. This may involve conducting experimental studies, controlling for confounding factors, and examining potential mechanisms through laboratory experiments or clinical trials. Causal relationships are typically established through a combination of evidence from different types of studies, replication of findings, and consensus among experts in the field.

Researchers and the scientific community need to communicate findings accurately, acknowledging the limitations of observational data and the need for further investigation. Additionally, critical evaluation and replication of research findings by independent researchers help strengthen the evidence base and provide a more comprehensive understanding of complex phenomena.

For example, if there's an observation of a positive correlation between smoking and having a stroke—meaning more strokes are seen in people who smoke—this's only a correlation at this point, indicating a statistical relationship between the two variables. However, a plausible explanation or mechanism linking the variables is necessary to establish an association.

In the case of smoking and stroke, if a sound explanation is proposed, such as the depletion of folate and subsequent increase in homocysteine levels promoting clot formation, it provides a potential pathway that links smoking to stroke. This association hypothesis can then be tested through further research, such as epidemiological studies or clinical trials, to examine if the proposed mechanism holds true and if there's evidence of a causal relationship.

199

The crucial step in scientific research is moving beyond correlation and conducting rigorous investigations to test the proposed associations. This involves designing studies that control for confounding factors, establishing temporal relationships, and examining dose-response relationships, among other considerations. By conducting well-designed studies and obtaining consistent and replicable results, researchers can provide more substantial evidence for the association and eventually establish it as a fact.

Scientists must go beyond observing correlations and strive to understand the underlying mechanisms and

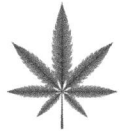

causal pathways. This deeper understanding allows for the development of more effective interventions, treatments, and preventive measures based on solid scientific evidence.

The Challenge of Going Against the Masses

When the general public holds strong beliefs or expectations about a particular treatment or solution, it can create difficulties for doctors in providing evidence-based recommendations that may contradict those beliefs. In an era where information is readily accessible, and opinions can spread quickly, there's a risk of misinformation or oversimplification of complex medical topics. This can lead to a situation where certain treatments or remedies, such as cannabis, are perceived as a panacea for a wide range of health issues.

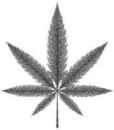

200

As healthcare professionals, doctors are responsible for basing their recommendations on scientific evidence and expertise. However, they must also navigate the delicate balance of respecting patient autonomy and addressing their concerns and preferences. Effective communication becomes crucial in such situations, as doctors must provide clear explanations, present the available evidence, and discuss potential risks and benefits associated with different treatment options.

While it can be challenging when public perception differs from medical consensus, doctors must maintain their commitment to evidence-based practice and continue educating their patients about the best available treatments. Building trust, providing comprehensive information, and engaging in open and honest conversations can help bridge the gap between public beliefs and medical expertise.

Acknowledging that self-medication can be risky and may lead to unintended consequences or interactions with other medications is crucial. It's always recommended to consult with qualified healthcare professionals before making treatment decisions.

A multifaceted approach is needed to address this issue, involving collaboration between politicians, businesses, medical professionals, and scientists. Here're a few key considerations:

- **Education and Awareness**: Enhancing public education and awareness about the potential risks of self-medication and the importance of seeking professional medical advice can empower individuals to make informed decisions about their health.
- **Accessible Healthcare**: Ensuring affordable and accessible healthcare services can help individuals obtain timely medical advice and appropriate treatments, reducing the need for self-medication.
- **Regulation and Oversight**: Implementing robust regulatory frameworks to monitor and evaluate the safety and efficacy of alternative remedies and treatments can help protect patients from unproven or potentially harmful interventions. This involves collaboration between regulatory authorities, medical professionals, and scientific experts.
- **Patient-Provider Communication**: Promoting effective communication between healthcare providers and patients is essential. Doctors should actively listen to patients, address their concerns, and provide clear explanations about treatment options, their benefits, and potential risks. This can help build trust and discourage patients from seeking unverified treatments.
- **Evidence-Based Practice**: Encouraging healthcare professionals to practice

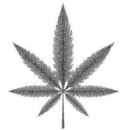

201

evidence-based medicine, which involves integrating the best available scientific evidence with clinical expertise and patient values, can ensure that patients receive treatments supported by rigorous research and have a higher likelihood of positive outcomes.

By addressing the root causes, promoting education, regulation, and effective communication, we can work toward a healthcare system that prioritizes patient safety, informed decision-making, and evidence-based care.

Building a sustainable healthcare system relies on the ethical conduct of all individuals involved, including healthcare professionals, researchers, policymakers, and patients. Ethical practices are essential for ensuring the safety and well-being of patients and the integrity of the healthcare system as a whole.

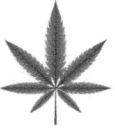

Regarding cannabis, it's true that there's still much we don't know about its potential benefits and risks. The unregulated use of cannabis can indeed be a cause for concern. While some studies suggest that cannabis may have therapeutic properties for some medical conditions, such as chronic pain or epilepsy, more research is needed to fully understand its effects, optimal dosages, and potential long-term consequences.

It's crucial to distinguish between the potential for treatment and the potential for abuse or adverse health effects when it comes to cannabis. This differentiation can help guide policies, regulations, and medical recommendations. By conducting rigorous scientific research and clinical trials, we can better understand cannabis's potential benefits and risks, allowing for evidence-based decision-making in healthcare.
Furthermore, effective regulation and oversight are necessary to ensure the safe and responsible use of

cannabis. This includes quality control measures, appropriate labelling and packaging, dosage guidelines, and restrictions on access for vulnerable populations, such as minors.

As our knowledge of cannabis evolves, we must remain open-minded, receptive to new evidence, and willing to adapt medical practices accordingly. Continued research, education, and responsible use are crucial to maximizing the potential benefits of cannabis while minimizing any potential harm.

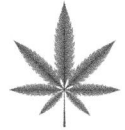

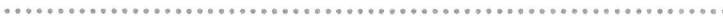

203

A woman went on a Caribbean cruise with a couple of friends. After a few days, she met Guy X and thought she had met "the one." The two had a good time for a few days, hardly spending time apart as they were getting to know each other.

Neither knew where this was headed, but they both hoped to make something big out of it. Around day ten, the woman couldn't locate her new love. She did her darnedest to find out where Guy X could have been, but had no luck. She was honest with herself about all possible outcomes from the beginning, including being ghosted. Yes, she was hurt, but she tried to forget about it. Her friends tried to cheer her up, but with only limited success.

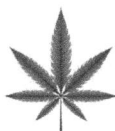

She then met Guy Y, who made her feel like all was going to be okay. Having spent a day with Guy Y, things were on fire, and the rebound seemed more certain. Was she cheating on Guy X at this point?

204

When the pair returned to her cabin for some quiet time, she received a call from Guy X. He told her that the ship had left him on one of the islands. He was sincere and willing to do anything to make it up to the woman that had made him cherish life again, and she understood.

After the call, would it have been cheating if she had continued with her "rebound" because it was too late to put the toothpaste back in the tube?

Bringing It All Together

For a drug we have known for decades, we should have tangible evidence of its uses, benefits, and effects before taking the issue lightly by giving it to anyone who asks for it. The leading causes of death in the developed world are cancer, heart disease, cerebrovascular disease (stroke), diabetes, and chronic lung disease. On the same turf, North America's four most common causes of disease are stress, cigarettes, alcohol, and substandard nutrition.

We've documented proof that cigarettes cause four of the five common causes of death. Cigarettes have been extensively studied, and their harmful effects on health, including their link to various diseases, are well-documented. Notably, it's not the nicotine in cigarettes causing health issues, but the smoke itself. This serves as a cautionary example of the importance of rigorous research and evidence-based decision-making regarding drugs.

Cannabis differs from tobacco in several ways, including its frequency of use and the presence of different active ingredients, such as THC and CBD. While cannabis has been used for medicinal and recreational purposes for centuries, our scientific knowledge about its potential benefits and risks is still evolving. Research has shown some promising therapeutic properties of cannabis, particularly in managing certain medical conditions like chronic pain, epilepsy, and chemotherapy-related nausea. However, further research is needed to fully understand its effects, proper dosing, potential interactions with other medications, and long-term consequences.

The composition of cannabis is complex, with numerous chemical compounds that may affect your body differently. It's crucial to conduct comprehensive research to identify and understand these components,

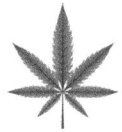

their individual effects, and any potential health implications associated with their use.

To ensure public health and safety, it's vital to approach cannabis use cautiously and follow evidence-based guidelines and regulations. This includes considerations of dosage, mode of administration, potential side effects, and appropriate use for specific medical conditions.
By continuing to invest in scientific research, we can gain a clearer understanding of the potential benefits and risks of cannabis, allowing for informed decision-making, responsible use, and the development of evidence-based guidelines for healthcare professionals and patients alike.

It's quite possible that smoking cannabis will share some of the same health complications as tobacco. However, it's too early to determine the pros and cons of cannabis in certain terms. The only thing we can do for now is find similarities between cannabis and tobacco. We can also deduce some of the effects of cannabis on the body based on what we know about tobacco. For example, both cannabis and tobacco are smoked, and we know the impact of smoke on the lungs and blood. We can then use that information to deduce associations between cannabis and the adverse health effects of inhaling it. Of course, the analyses must adjust for the differences in the quantity of smoke and frequency of smoking tobacco instead of cannabis. By drawing parallels and considering the existing knowledge about tobacco smoke, we can make some inferences about the potential health implications of cannabis smoke.

Inhaling any smoke, whether from tobacco or cannabis, can introduce harmful substances into the respiratory system. Combustion generates various toxic compounds, such as carbon monoxide, tar, and particulate matter, which can irritate your lungs and contribute to respiratory issues. Prolonged exposure

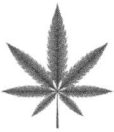

to these substances has been associated with an increased risk of developing chronic bronchitis, COPD, and other respiratory conditions.

It's worth noting that the quantity and frequency of smoke inhalation differ between tobacco and cannabis use. Generally, cannabis smokers smoke less frequently and in smaller amounts than tobacco smokers. However, further research is still needed to better understand the specific risks associated with cannabis smoke and its potential long-term effects on respiratory health.
Additionally, it's essential to consider alternative methods of cannabis consumption that don't involve smoking, such as vaporization, edibles, or **tinctures**. These methods may offer potential benefits in reducing exposure to harmful combustion byproducts associated with smoking.

As our understanding of cannabis continues to evolve, ongoing research is crucial to assess the potential risks and benefits associated with its use, particularly in relation to different modes of consumption. By studying the effects of cannabis on the body and conducting comparative analyses with tobacco, we can gather valuable insights and develop evidence-based guidelines to minimize potential health risks.

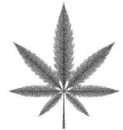

207

The Fundamental Principles in Medicine

While "do no harm" is often considered a fundamental principle, it's not interpreted as an absolute prohibition against causing any harm to patients. Instead, it's understood in the context of the overall benefit that medical interventions can provide.

In medical practice, the goal is to maximize the overall benefit to the patient while minimizing the potential harm or risk associated with a particular treatment. Healthcare professionals carefully assess various interventions' potential risks and benefits and make informed decisions based on the available evidence and the individual patient's circumstances.

Certain medical interventions, such as prescribing medications or performing surgeries, inherently involve some level of risk or harm. However, the critical consideration is whether the expected benefits of the intervention outweigh the potential risks and harm. Medical professionals strive to achieve the best possible patient outcomes by carefully evaluating the balance between potential benefits and risks.

In this risk-benefit assessment, factors such as the severity of the condition, the available alternative treatments, the patient's overall health, and their personal preferences and values are taken into account. The aim is to provide treatments with a favourable risk-benefit ratio, where the benefits outweigh the potential harm.

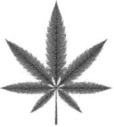

208

While medical interventions involve an inherent level of risk, it's essential to remember that healthcare professionals strive to act in their patients' best interests and make decisions based on sound medical knowledge, ethical principles, and each patient's individual circumstances.

This brings us to the most fundamental principle in medicine: **patient autonomy**. Patient autonomy recognizes the right of individuals to make decisions about their own healthcare based on their own values, preferences, and understanding of the relevant information.

Informed consent is an essential component of respecting patient autonomy. Before undergoing any medical treatment or procedure, patients have the right to be provided with clear and accurate information about the nature of the treatment, its purpose, potential benefits, risks, and any available alternatives.

This enables patients to understand the implications of their choices and make autonomous decisions.

When it comes to cannabis use, education and informed decision-making are crucial. Patients should have access to reliable and unbiased information about cannabis, including its potential benefits, risks, side effects, and interactions with other medications. Healthcare professionals are essential in providing this information and guiding patients toward evidence-based decisions.

By providing accurate and comprehensive information, healthcare professionals can empower patients to make informed choices about their healthcare, including the use of cannabis. This involves discussing the potential benefits and risks, addressing any concerns or misconceptions, and helping patients weigh the available evidence in the context of their individual health conditions and goals.

Healthcare professionals must stay updated on the latest research and evidence regarding cannabis to provide accurate information and guidance to patients. Open and honest communication between healthcare providers and patients fosters trust, encourages shared decision-making, and respects patient autonomy.

209

Amidst all the commotion, we still want to restore the therapeutic alliance because that creates a sustainable healthcare system. A solid therapeutic alliance is essential for effective healthcare delivery and positive health outcomes. When patients trust and feel supported by their healthcare providers, they're more likely to actively participate in their own care, follow treatment plans, and make informed decisions about their health. This improves treatment adherence, outcomes, and overall patient satisfaction.

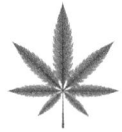

To restore and strengthen the therapeutic alliance, healthcare providers must listen to their patients, respect their autonomy, and involve them in decision-making. Open and honest communication, empathy, and a patient-centred approach are critical elements of fostering a strong therapeutic alliance.

Ultimately, a healthcare system that not only focuses on emergencies and chronic illnesses, but also promotes healthier lives is essential for the population's well-being. This requires a collaborative effort between healthcare providers, policymakers, and the community to prioritize preventive care, health education, and interventions aimed at promoting overall health and well-being.

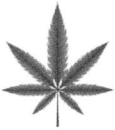

Imagine you have a mechanic who works on your car. One day you think the mechanic's job is too mundane, and you could fix the car yourself anytime. Without mechanical knowledge and understanding, you're almost certain to do more damage to your vehicle. This'll cost you more if you take it to the same mechanic to fix the problems you created. It's wrong for a mechanic to take advantage of you, but that's not a reason to do the job yourself.

A similar relationship exists between doctors and patients, which is the basis of our healthcare system. When one doctor doesn't work, it's not a reason to start self-medicating, as you're more likely to cost yourself more in the long run. A more prudent way to deal with this situation is to seek a second opinion or look for another primary care doctor. At no point should self-medicating be acceptable, yet our society has embraced this idea.

Self-medicating without proper knowledge and guidance from healthcare professionals can be risky and potentially lead to adverse health effects. While it's essential to trust the medical system and seek appropriate medical care, being an informed and proactive patient is also crucial.

Engaging in self-medication without the necessary expertise and guidance can have serious consequences, including misdiagnosis, ineffective treatments, medication interactions, and delays in receiving appropriate care. It's crucial to rely on the expertise of healthcare professionals who have undergone extensive training and have the knowledge and experience to provide proper medical advice and treatment.

One of the biggest problems with cannabis is the legal problems that may run for as long as they have haunted the tobacco industry. Things are more likely to get more complicated with cannabis than we have seen with tobacco. For reasons already explained, the benefits of cannabis are mainly speculative, and some of the effects can be unpredictable. As cannabis legalization and regulation continue to evolve, various legal considerations need to be addressed, including issues related to production, distribution, sales, advertising, and consumer protection.

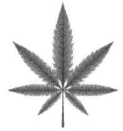

211

Additionally, the benefits and potential risks of cannabis use are still being studied and understood. While evidence suggests that cannabis may have therapeutic properties for certain medical conditions, the research is ongoing, and there're still many unknowns. The effects of cannabis can vary from person to person due to factors such as individual physiology, metabolism, and genetic makeup.

Various factors, including body weight, body fat percentage, liver function, frequency and duration of use, and the method of consumption, influence the duration of cannabis in your body. Depending on these factors, THC can be detected in your body for varying lengths of time, ranging from days to weeks. However, it's important to note that the presence of

THC in your body doesn't necessarily equate to impairment, as THC can remain detectable long after its psychoactive effects have worn off.

As the understanding of cannabis and its effects continues to advance, it's crucial to have comprehensive and evidence-based regulations in place to address legal, medical, and public health considerations. This includes education and awareness programs to help individuals make informed decisions about cannabis use and to promote responsible and safe consumption practices.

The Legal Conundrum: Cannabis and Impaired Driving

The legal status of cannabis has been a subject of much debate and discussion. One area that raises significant concerns is impaired driving under the influence of cannabis. Let's explore the complexities surrounding the legal implications of cannabis use and impaired driving, shedding light on the challenges faced by the legal system.

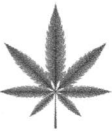

212

1. **Legal Status and Impaired Driving**: Currently, if a person is found to be intoxicated with an illegal drug while committing a crime, the legal consequences are often severe. However, the situation becomes more intricate when the drug in question is legal, such as cannabis. Let's consider the scenario of a drunk driver who tragically hits a pedestrian. In many jurisdictions, this would likely result in a prison sentence. However, the legal outcome might differ if the driver was not under the influence of any illegal substances.
2. **The Cannabis Dilemma**: When it comes to cannabis, the issue becomes even more complex. If cannabis is illegal, a driver impaired by cannabis who causes a

fatal accident will face strict legal consequences. However, if cannabis is legalized and regulated, uncertainties arise. Determining impairment levels due to cannabis use becomes challenging, as the effects of cannabis on driving performance can vary depending on various factors.

3. **Understanding Impairment and Cannabis Use**: Cannabis contains THC, which can affect cognitive and motor functions. The impairment caused by cannabis use can include slowed reaction time, altered perception, impaired coordination, and decreased attention. These effects can have serious implications for driving safety.

4. **The Science Behind Impairment**: Scientific studies have shown that cannabis use can impair driving performance and increase the risk of accidents. However, unlike alcohol, there's currently no consensus on specific legal limits for THC levels in your bloodstream that equate to impairment. The effects of cannabis on individuals can vary due to factors such as tolerance, frequency of use, and individual metabolism.

213

5. **Navigating the Legal Maze**: Determining impairment caused by cannabis use poses significant challenges for law enforcement and legal authorities. The lack of standardized tests and established thresholds for impairment make it difficult to establish clear legal guidelines. Additionally, detecting recent cannabis use is more complex than alcohol testing, as THC can remain detectable in bodily fluids long after impairment has subsided.

6. **Moving Forward**: Addressing the legal complexities of cannabis and impaired driving requires a multifaceted approach. Continued research is necessary to

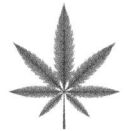

establish evidence-based impairment standards
and develop reliable testing methods.
Public education and awareness campaigns
are crucial to informing individuals about
the potential risks of cannabis use
and driving impairment.

The legal landscape surrounding cannabis and impaired driving is complex and evolving. Balancing
public safety and individual rights presents significant
challenges for the legal system. Ongoing research, informed policy decisions, and effective education are
essential to ensure road safety and minimize the risks
associated with cannabis use and impaired driving.

Legal limit for the blood-cannabis level

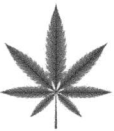

Setting a general legal limit for cannabis impairment,
similar to alcohol, is challenging due to the differences in how the substances are processed and detected in your body. Unlike alcohol, which is metabolized
relatively quickly and can be measured in your blood,
cannabis compounds, notably THC, can remain detectable in bodily tissues for an extended period.

214

The presence of THC in your blood doesn't necessarily
correspond to current impairment at the time of an
incident. THC can be detected in your blood even days
after consumption, making it difficult to accurately
determine the timing and degree of impairment. This
poses a significant hurdle when establishing a standard legal blood cannabis level for determining impairment.
Additionally, individual factors, such as tolerance,
frequency of use, and metabolism, can influence the
effects of cannabis on an individual's impairment,
further complicating the establishment of universal
standards. A person who consumed cannabis several
days ago may still have THC in their blood, but their
impairment level may be minimal compared to someone who consumed cannabis more recently.

Given these challenges, current approaches to addressing cannabis-related impaired driving focus on field sobriety tests and drug recognition evaluations conducted by trained law enforcement officers. These assessments aim to evaluate observable signs of impairment, such as impaired coordination, balance, and cognitive function, rather than relying solely on blood cannabis levels.

It's crucial to continue research efforts to develop reliable methods for assessing cannabis impairment, considering the dose, frequency of use, and the specific effects of different cannabis strains. Such research can help inform policy decisions and create a more nuanced approach to addressing cannabis impairment and ensuring road safety.

Cannabis and the legal challenges

The legal status of cannabis varies across different jurisdictions, and its consequences can also differ. In some cases, individuals may exploit legal loopholes or uncertainties to their advantage, creating challenges for law enforcement and the justice system.

215

It's essential to approach the analysis of social problems related to widespread cannabis use with caution. Drawing direct comparisons between different countries or social settings can be complex due to the numerous factors that influence outcomes. Each context has its unique cultural, legal, and socio-economic considerations, which can significantly impact the effects of cannabis use and associated social issues.

Furthermore, it's essential to differentiate between correlations and objective associations when evaluating the effects of cannabis. Correlation simply indicates a statistical relationship between two variables, but it doesn't necessarily imply causation or provide a comprehensive understanding of the underlying mechanisms. To establish objective as-

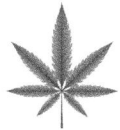

sociations, rigorous scientific research is needed, taking into account various factors such as dosage, frequency of use, individual differences, and potential confounding variables.

Given the evolving nature of cannabis research, it's crucial to continue conducting studies that adhere to scientific principles and methodology. These studies can help establish reliable, evidence-based knowledge, which can then inform policy decisions, regulatory frameworks, and public understanding of the potential benefits and risks associated with cannabis use.

Irresponsible application of numbers is like tossing a lit candle into a pool of gasoline; throwing something relatively harmless into a highly volatile environment. Irrespective of the reason for throwing the candle, the result of tossing it in the gasoline pool will have serve consequences.

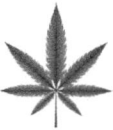

216

Regarding the widespread use of cannabis, it's vital to consider the potential ramifications on various levels: personal, economic, political, and social. While there may be arguments in favour of encouraging cannabis use for different purposes, it's crucial to assess the potential risks and unintended consequences that could arise.

Understanding the impact of widespread cannabis use requires careful consideration of various factors. These include potential health risks, productivity and economic stability effects, regulatory challenges, social implications, and the balance between individual liberties and public welfare.

To make informed decisions, policymakers and society as a whole should draw upon rigorous scientific research, comprehensive data analysis, and evidence-based evaluations. This approach helps minimize the likelihood of exacerbating existing problems or creating new ones while addressing the concerns and needs of individuals and communities.

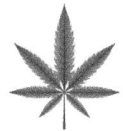

So What?

In today's society, there's a concerning trend of disregarding scientific principles and knowledge in favour of immediate gratification and simplified explanations. This erosion of intellectual curiosity and patience for understanding complex concepts threatens the very principles that have guided and protected us throughout history.

The foundations of scientific inquiry are built upon the tireless pursuit of knowledge, the questioning of established ideas, and the willingness to delve into the intricacies of various fields. However, in a world where superficial understanding and quick fixes are favoured over in-depth exploration, we risk losing the essence of scientific progress and critical thinking.

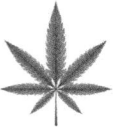

218

It's essential to recognize the value of scientific education and its role in shaping our understanding of the world. Merely relying on introductory science classes from high school or accepting oversimplified explanations without seeking deeper insights can lead to misguided conclusions and a distorted view of reality.

To safeguard the principles that have propelled us forward, we must foster a renewed appreciation for science and its intricate complexities. This entails promoting scientific literacy, encouraging a spirit of inquiry, and embracing the patience and perseverance required to uncover meaningful insights.

Ultimately, the pursuit of knowledge should transcend generations, bridging the gap between past discoveries and future advancements. By nurturing a culture that values scientific exploration and critical thinking, we can counteract the current trend and ensure that our understanding of the world continues to evolve and thrive.

In the past, scientists were revered as leaders who guided society into the realm of the unknown, driven by a desire to help people understand the world they live in. The pursuit of knowledge and the dissemination of accurate information were paramount. However, in today's world, there's a shift where the focus has shifted toward pleasing people and telling them what they want to hear rather than presenting objective and evidence-based findings.

Science isn't about catering to individual preferences or confirming preconceived beliefs. It's about seeking the truth and providing a reliable understanding of the natural world. Ignorance, unfortunately, has gained prominence in some communities, undermining our collective progress and weakening our ability to make informed decisions as a species.

Attempting to educate someone who staunchly refuses to acknowledge or seek knowledge is akin to trying to dry oneself while swimming in water. It's a futile endeavour. Just as water will keep us wet, those who proudly embrace ignorance will turn a deaf ear to information and resist opportunities for growth and understanding. This makes the efforts of scientists and educators fruitless in such circumstances.

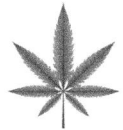

219

Nevertheless, scientists and educators must remain steadfast in their dedication to knowledge and the pursuit of truth. Their role is to continue conducting rigorous research, sharing reliable information, and promoting critical thinking. While it may be challenging to reach those who are resistant to knowledge, disseminating accurate information can still positively impact those who are open-minded and willing to engage in meaningful dialogue.

By valuing and supporting scientific inquiry, promoting evidence-based reasoning, and fostering a culture of intellectual curiosity, we can work towards reversing the current trend of ignorance and ensure that

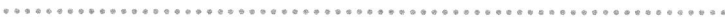

knowledge and understanding prevail for the betterment of society as a whole.

Scientifically speaking, cannabis is a relatively understudied and complex plant. While it has been used for various purposes throughout history, our understanding of its effects on the human body and mind is still evolving. It's vital to approach cannabis scientifically, exploring its potential benefits and risks and presenting accurate information to the world.

To truly understand cannabis, we must conduct rigorous research that encompasses various aspects, including its chemical composition, pharmacological properties, potential therapeutic applications, and potential risks. This scientific exploration will provide us with valuable insights into the effects of cannabis consumption in all its forms.

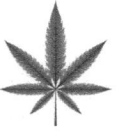

Promoting cannabis without a comprehensive understanding of its effects would be irresponsible and could potentially lead to unintended consequences. Gathering scientific evidence and data to inform decision-making, public health policies, and responsible use is crucial.

By conducting scientific studies and research, we can uncover the true nature of cannabis, its potential benefits, and any potential adverse effects. This knowledge will empower individuals, policymakers, and healthcare professionals to make informed decisions regarding its use, regulation, and potential societal impact.

It's important to emphasize that scientific exploration of cannabis shouldn't be dismissed or delayed. Waiting to explore cannabis until after its widespread promotion could lead to missed opportunities for understanding and addressing potential risks and harnessing its potential benefits.

Ultimately, society should have access to accurate and comprehensive information about cannabis, enabling individuals to make informed choices based on their own values and priorities. By approaching cannabis with scientific rigour, we can ensure a well-informed public discourse and promote responsible use while maximizing the potential benefits and minimizing potential harms.

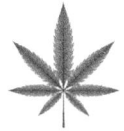

Glossary

11-hydroxy-THC: A metabolite of THC, the active compound in cannabis.

Acetylcholine: A neurotransmitter involved in muscle control and other functions.

Action potential: A brief electrical signal travelling along a nerve cell's membrane.

Addiction: A complex condition characterized by compulsive substance use despite negative consequences.

Adenocarcinoma: A type of cancer that begins in glandular cells, often occurring in the lungs.

Adenosine triphosphate (ATP): A molecule that stores and releases energy for cellular processes.

Agitation: Restlessness and emotional distress.

Alcohol dehydrogenase: An enzyme breaking down alcohol in the body.

Alcohol: A psychoactive substance affecting the central nervous system.

Alternative medicine: Non-traditional approaches to healthcare.

223

Alveolar membrane: The thin barrier between alveoli and capillaries where gas exchange occurs.

Alveolus: Tiny air sacs in the lungs where oxygen is exchanged for carbon dioxide during respiration.

Alzheimer's disease: A progressive neurological disorder causing memory loss and cognitive decline.

Amino acid: A building block of proteins and essential for various bodily functions.

Amphetamines: Stimulant drugs that increase alertness and energy.

Analgesic: Pain-relieving substance or medication that alleviates pain without causing loss of consciousness.

Anecdotal evidence: Informal, non-scientific observations or personal experiences that may not be representative or reliable for drawing conclusions.

Angle-closure glaucoma: A less common form of glaucoma caused by a narrow angle between the cornea and iris.

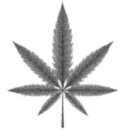

Anti-inflammatory: Substance that reduces inflammation, which is the body's response to injury or infection.

Antibodies: Proteins produced by the immune system to identify and neutralize harmful substances.

Anticoagulation: Preventing blood clot formation.

Antidepressants: Medications used to alleviate symptoms of depression.

Antioxidant: A molecule that helps protect cells from damage caused by free radicals.

Antipsychotic medication: Drugs used to manage symptoms of psychosis and related disorders.

Anxiety: A mental state characterized by excessive worry, fear, or nervousness. Cannabis use may impact anxiety levels, with some individuals experiencing increased anxiety as a side effect.

Anxiolytic drugs: Medications used to alleviate anxiety and promote a sense of calm.

Anxious: Feeling worried, nervous, or uneasy.

Anxious: Feeling worried, uneasy, or apprehensive.

Aqueous humour: The clear fluid filling the space in the front of the eye.

224

Aspirin: A medication often used to reduce pain, inflammation, and fever, and prevent blood clots.

Atherosclerosis: Buildup of plaque in arteries, a leading cause of cardiovascular disease.

Attention deficit disorder: A condition characterized by difficulty focusing and controlling impulses.

Attention deficit hyperactivity disorder: A neurodevelopmental disorder marked by inattention, hyperactivity, and impulsivity.

Autism spectrum disorders: Range of developmental conditions affecting social and communication skills.

Autism: A developmental disorder characterized by challenges in social interaction and communication.

Autoimmune disorder: A condition where the immune system attacks healthy cells.

Axons: Long projections of neurons that transmit electrical impulses to other cells.

Barbiturates: A class of sedative medications that de-

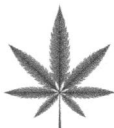

press the central nervous system.

Benzene: A chemical compound found in tobacco smoke and other pollutants, known to be carcinogenic.

Benzodiazepines: Medications that induce relaxation and reduce anxiety by enhancing the effects of a neurotransmitter called GABA.

Beta receptors: Proteins on cell surfaces that respond to certain neurotransmitters and hormones.

Binary fission: A type of cell division seen in bacteria and some other single-celled organisms.

Biochemical ingredients: The chemical compounds present in a substance, in this case, cannabis, that contribute to its effects.

Biochemical reactions: Chemical processes occurring within cells to maintain life.

Bipolar disorder: A mood disorder characterized by alternating periods of depression and mania.

Blood alcohol concentration: Amount of alcohol in the bloodstream.

Blood cannabis levels: Concentration of cannabis components in the bloodstream.

Blood clots: Clumps of blood cells that can obstruct blood vessels.

225

Blood volume: The total amount of blood in the circulatory system.

Blood-brain barrier: A protective barrier between the bloodstream and the brain, regulating the passage of substances.

Blurred vision: Reduced clarity of vision, often making objects appear unfocused.

Body mass index: A measure of body weight relative to height.

Bone marrow: Soft tissue found within bones responsible for producing blood cells.

Brain chemistry: Chemical processes in the brain influencing behaviour and mental state.

Brain's reward system: Neural circuitry involved in pleasure and reinforcement.

Bronchi: The two main air passages leading from the trachea to the lungs, branching into smaller bronchioles.

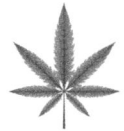

Bronchial constriction: Narrowing of the airways, making breathing difficult.

Bronchiectasis: A condition in which the airways become damaged and widened.

Bronchioles: Small airway branches in the lungs connecting bronchi to alveoli.

Bronchitis: Inflammation of the bronchi, often caused by infections or irritants, leading to coughing, mucus production, and difficulty breathing.

Bronchodilators: Medications that relax the muscles in the airways, improving airflow.

Cancer: A group of diseases characterized by uncontrolled cell growth and the potential to invade other tissues.

Cannabinoid receptors: Receptors in the body's endocannabinoid system that interacts with cannabinoids, influencing various physiological functions.

Cannabis-induced Psychosis: Psychotic symptoms triggered by cannabis use.

Cannabis: Cannabis, commonly known as marijuana or weed, is a plant that contains various compounds, including cannabinoids like THC and CBD. It has been used for both medicinal and recreational purposes.

Carcinogens: Substances that can cause cancer.

Cardiovascular health: The overall health of the heart and blood vessels.

Catatonia: A state of immobility or unresponsiveness.

CB1 receptors: Receptors in the endocannabinoid system found in the brain and nervous system that interact with cannabinoids like THC.

CBD (Cannabidiol): A non-psychoactive compound found in cannabis with potential therapeutic effects, such as anti-inflammatory, analgesic, and anti-anxiety properties.

Cellular metabolism: Chemical processes within cells that produce energy and result in the exchange of gases at the cellular level.

Central nervous system: The brain and spinal cord, controlling most body functions.

Central vision: The ability to see fine details and focus on objects directly in front of the eyes.

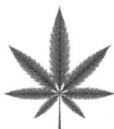

Cervix: The lower, narrow part of the uterus connecting to the vagina.

Chest pain: Discomfort or pain in the chest often associated with heart issues.

Chronic Bronchiolitis: Inflammation of the bronchioles, causing breathing difficulties.

Chronic bronchitis: A type of chronic obstructive pulmonary disease (COPD) characterized by persistent inflammation of the bronchi and excessive mucus production.

Chronic hypoxia: Long-term deficiency of oxygen supply to tissues.

Chronic inflammation: Persistent inflammation that can contribute to various health issues.

Chronic Obstructive Pulmonary Diseases (COPD): A group of progressive lung diseases that obstruct airflow.

Chronic pain: Persistent or long-lasting pain that persists beyond the normal healing time and often requires ongoing management.

Chronic respiratory problems: Long-term conditions affecting the lungs and airways, often leading to breathing difficulties.

Ciliary muscle: A muscle that controls the shape of the lens in the eye, affecting focus.

227

Clear cell carcinoma: A type of cancer characterized by clear cells and occurring in various organs.

Clotting events: The formation of blood clots.

Clotting factors: Substances in the blood involved in the blood clotting process.

Cocaine: A stimulant drug that affects the central nervous system.

Cognition: Mental processes related to acquiring knowledge, perception, memory, and problem-solving.

Cognitive deficits: Impairments in cognitive functions, such as memory, attention, and problem-solving.

Cognitive function: Mental processes related to learning, memory, problem-solving, and decision-making.

Cognitive impairment: Decline in cognitive function,

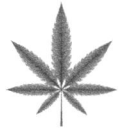

including memory and thinking abilities.

Columnar epithelial cells: Cells with a taller, elongated shape that line the gastrointestinal tract and other structures.

Combustion: The process of burning, which produces heat and usually involves the release of gases and particles.

Conception: The fertilization of an egg by a sperm, initiating pregnancy.

Confounding factors: Variables that can impact the relationship between two variables being studied.

Coordination: The ability to move body parts smoothly and efficiently.

Coping mechanisms: Strategies and behaviours used to deal with stress and challenges.

Cornea: The clear front part of the eye that covers the iris and pupil.

Coronary arteries: Blood vessels supplying oxygen and nutrients to the heart muscle.

Cravings: Intense desires to use a substance.

Cyanosis: Bluish discoloration of the skin and mucous membranes due to low oxygen levels.

Cytochrome P450: A group of enzymes metabolizing many medications.

Delirium tremens: Severe alcohol withdrawal symptoms, including hallucinations and seizures.

Delusions: False beliefs that persist despite evidence to the contrary.

Dementia: A general term for a decline in cognitive ability affecting daily life.

Dependence: Physical or psychological reliance on a substance, often resulting in withdrawal symptoms upon discontinuation.

Depolarization: A change in the electrical charge of a neuron, leading to the firing of an action potential.

Depression: A mood disorder characterized by persistent sadness, loss of interest or pleasure, and other emotional and physical symptoms.

Detoxify: The process of removing toxins or harmful substances from the body.

Diabetes mellitus: A chronic metabolic disorder

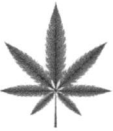

characterized by high blood sugar levels.

Diarrhea: Frequent and loose bowel movements.

Diethylstilbestrol: A synthetic estrogen once prescribed to pregnant women, linked to health issues in offspring.

Diffusion: The movement of molecules from an area of higher concentration to an area of lower concentration.

Digestion: The process of breaking down food in the gastrointestinal tract to extract nutrients and energy.

Disordered thinking: Unorganized and illogical thought patterns.

Divergent thinking: A thought process that generates creative ideas by exploring various possibilities.

DNA: Genetic material that carries instructions for the development and functioning of living organisms.

Dopamine: A neurotransmitter associated with pleasure, reward, and motivation.

Dose: The amount of a substance, such as cannabis, taken at one time, often used to measure medication or drug intake.

Down syndrome: A genetic disorder caused by the presence of an extra chromosome 21, resulting in developmental delays and characteristic features.

229

Dravet syndrome: A rare genetic epilepsy disorder causing frequent, prolonged seizures.

Drooping: Sagging or hanging down of body parts, often referring to eyelids.

Drug dependence: A physiological or psychological need for a substance.

Drug reservoirs: Sites where drugs can accumulate in the body.

Drug-drug interactions: Effects when one medication influences the actions of another.

Dysplasia: Abnormal cell growth that may lead to cancer if not treated.

Edibles: Food products infused with cannabis extracts, often used for their slower and longer-lasting effects compared to smoking or vaping.

Ego: In Freudian psychology, the part of the psyche mediating between the id and superego.

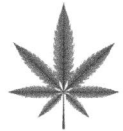

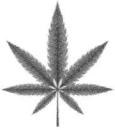

Emphysema: A type of COPD characterized by damage to the air sacs in the lungs.

Endocannabinoid system: A complex system of receptors and molecules that regulates various processes in the body, including mood, pain, and appetite.

Endorphins: Natural chemicals produced by the brain that contribute to feelings of pleasure and pain relief.

Endothelial cells: Cells lining blood vessels, including the walls of capillaries, where gas exchange between blood and tissues occurs.

Enzyme activities: Rates at which enzymes facilitate chemical reactions.

Enzyme induction: Increase in enzyme production due to drug exposure.

Enzymes: Proteins that facilitate chemical reactions in the body.

Epidiolex: A medication containing CBD used to treat seizures associated with Lennox-Gastaut syndrome and Dravet syndrome.

Epilepsy: A neurological disorder characterized by recurrent seizures.

Epithelial cells: Cells that form the surface of tissues and organs, serving protective and absorptive functions.

Erectile dysfunction: Inability to achieve or maintain an erection sufficient for sexual activity.

Erection: The process of engorgement and enlargement of the penis due to increased blood flow.

Erythromycin: An antibiotic inhibiting bacterial growth.

Essential fatty acids: Unsaturated fats necessary for bodily function but not synthesized by the body.

Estrogen: A female hormone with various roles, including regulating the menstrual cycle.

Ethical: Pertaining to moral principles and values.

Euphoria: A feeling of intense happiness, often associated with the use of certain substances.

Euphoric effect: A feeling of intense happiness or pleasure.

Evidence-based approaches: Decision-making based on scientific research and well-established evidence rather than personal beliefs or anecdotal accounts.

External Respiration: The exchange of oxygen and carbon dioxide between the lungs and the external environment.

Fat-soluble drug: A medication that dissolves in fat and is stored in body fat.

Fat-soluble: Capable of dissolving in fats or lipids.

Fetal alcohol syndrome: A condition resulting from maternal alcohol consumption during pregnancy, leading to developmental and intellectual issues in the fetus.

Fetal life: The period of development from conception to birth.

Fetus: The developing human organism after the embryonic stage and before birth.

Folate: A B-vitamin essential for DNA synthesis and cell division.

Formaldehyde: A toxic compound found in various products, including tobacco smoke and building materials.

Free radicals: Unstable molecules that can cause oxidative damage to cells and DNA.

Gamma-aminobutyric acid: An inhibitory neurotransmitter that regulates brain activity.

Gaseous exchange: The process of exchanging gases (oxygen and carbon dioxide) between the blood and air in the lungs.

Genetic makeup: An individual's unique combination of genes inherited from their parents.

Genetic mutations: Changes in DNA sequences that can lead to altered gene function.

Genetic predisposition: A person's increased likelihood of developing a particular condition due to their genetic makeup.

Genetics: The study of inherited traits and genetic variation.

Glaucoma: A group of eye conditions characterized by damage to the optic nerve, often associated with increased intraocular pressure.

Glutamate: A major excitatory neurotransmitter in the brain.

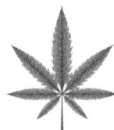

Government regulations: Laws and rules established by governing bodies to manage the legal production, distribution, and use of substances like cannabis.

Hallucinations: False sensory perceptions that seem real.

Halos: Rings of light that may appear around bright objects, often a symptom of certain eye conditions.

Healthcare providers: Individuals and institutions offering medical services, including diagnosis, treatment, and prevention of illnesses.

Heart attacks: Damage to the heart muscle due to blocked blood flow.

Heart failure: A condition in which the heart is unable to pump blood effectively.

Hemoglobin: Protein in red blood cells that binds to oxygen for transport in the blood.

Herb: In the context of cannabis, it refers to the dried leaves, flowers, or other parts of the plant used for various purposes.

Hippocampus: A region of the brain involved in memory formation and learning.

Homocysteine: An amino acid associated with cardiovascular disease risk.

Hormones: Chemical messengers produced by glands that regulate various bodily functions and processes.

Hydrochloric acid: A strong acid found in the stomach that aids in digestion.

Hydrophilic heads: The water-attracting part of a phospholipid molecule.

Hydrophobic tails: The water-repelling part of a phospholipid molecule.

Hyperhomocysteinemia: Elevated levels of homocysteine in the blood.

Hypertension: High blood pressure, a risk factor for various cardiovascular issues.

Hypoxia: Insufficient oxygen supply to body tissues.

Id: In Freudian psychology, the primitive and impulsive part of the psyche.

Immunizations: Medical interventions to enhance immunity against infectious diseases.

Impaired coordination: Reduced ability to control

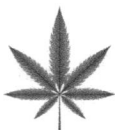

body movements accurately.
Impaired motor coordination: Decreased ability to control body movements effectively.
Increased intraocular pressure: Elevated pressure within the eye, a major risk factor for glaucoma.
Infertility: Inability to conceive or carry a pregnancy to term.
Inflammation: A physiological response of the body to injury or infection, characterized by redness, swelling, pain, and heat. In the context of cannabis, some compounds like CBD are believed to have anti-inflammatory properties.
Insomnia: Difficulty falling asleep or staying asleep.
Insulator: A material that restricts the flow of electricity.
Intellect: Mental capacity for understanding and reasoning.
Intellectual capacity: The overall cognitive ability to process information, solve problems, and learn.
Intellectual impairment: Deficits in cognitive functioning, affecting learning and problem-solving.
Internal Respiration: The exchange of gases between the bloodstream and body tissues.
Iris: The coloured part of the eye that controls the size of the pupil.

233

Irritability: Easily provoked or frustrated state of mind.
Lennox-Gastaut syndrome: A severe form of epilepsy characterized by multiple types of seizures.
Lens: The transparent structure in the eye that focuses light onto the retina.
Leydig cells: Cells in the testes that produce testosterone.
Lightheaded: Feeling dizzy or faint.
Lipid bilayer: A double layer of lipid molecules that forms the basis of cell membranes.
Longitudinal studies: Research conducted over an extended period to analyze changes and trends over time.
Lung architecture: The structural arrangement of lung tissues and airways.

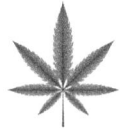

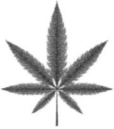

Lung cancer: Cancer that originates in the lungs, often linked to smoking and exposure to carcinogens.

Medical advice: Recommendations provided by healthcare professionals to address health concerns and guide treatment decisions.

Medical conditions: Health issues or illnesses that require medical attention, diagnosis, and treatment.

Medical professionals: Licensed healthcare practitioners, such as doctors and nurses, who diagnose, treat, and manage medical conditions.

Medicinal cannabis: Cannabis used for therapeutic purposes to treat or manage medical conditions.

Menstrual blood loss: The amount of blood lost during menstruation.

Metabolic processes: Chemical reactions in the body that convert food into energy and support growth, maintenance, and other functions.

Metabolism: The chemical processes that convert food into energy and support various bodily functions.

Metabolites: Molecules resulting from metabolic processes.

Metaplasia: A reversible change in cell type, often due to irritation or stress.

234

Methionine: An essential amino acid involved in various biochemical processes.

Methyl folate: A biologically active form of folate.

Missed period: Absence of menstruation, often indicating pregnancy.

Mitochondria: Cellular organelles responsible for producing energy (ATP) through cellular respiration.

Mood regulation: The ability to manage and stabilize emotions.

Mood-altering medications: Drugs that can affect emotional states and behaviours.

Moral: Relating to principles of right and wrong conduct.

Morning sickness: Nausea and vomiting experienced during early pregnancy.

Multiple sclerosis: An autoimmune disorder affecting the central nervous system's myelin.

Muscle aches: Pain or discomfort in muscles.

Muscle mass: The amount of muscle tissue in the body.

Myelin sheath: A protective layer around nerve fibres, enhancing signal transmission.

Myelin: A fatty substance that insulates axons, allowing for faster nerve impulse transmission.

Myelination: The process of forming a protective sheath (myelin) around nerve fibres.

Myocardial infarction: A heart attack, resulting from blocked blood flow to the heart muscle.

Nausea: A sensation of sickness or discomfort often associated with a feeling of needing to vomit.

Nerve impulse transmission: The propagation of electrical signals along nerve cells.

Nerve signalling: Transmission of signals between nerve cells, enabling communication in the nervous system.

Neural circuitry: The complex interconnected pathways of neurons in the brain and nervous system.

Neurobehavioral development: The combined growth of neurological and behavioural aspects during development.

Neurochemical signalling: Transmission of information in the nervous system through the release and binding of chemicals (neurotransmitters).

235

Neuronal activity: Electrical impulses and chemical signals generated by nerve cells (neurons) in the nervous system.

Neurons: Specialized cells transmitting electrical and chemical signals in the nervous system.

Neuroprotective: Properties that help protect nerve cells from damage.

Neuropsychiatry: A field of medicine studying the relationship between brain function and psychiatric disorders.

Neuroscience: The scientific study of the nervous system and its functions.

Neurotransmitters: Chemical messengers that transmit signals between nerve cells in the brain and body.

Neurotransmitters: Chemical messengers that

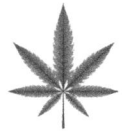

transmit signals between nerve cells.

Nicotine: A highly addictive chemical found in tobacco products.

Non-specific symptoms: Signs that are not clearly associated with a specific condition.

Norepinephrine: A neurotransmitter influencing attention, mood, and stress response.

Norepinephrine: A neurotransmitter that affects attention, alertness, and stress response.

Norepinephrine: A neurotransmitter that plays a role in the body's "fight or flight" response to stress.

Numbness: Loss of sensation or feeling in a body part.

Nutritional deficiencies: Lack of essential nutrients needed for proper bodily function.

Obsessive-compulsive disorder: A mental disorder characterized by unwanted repetitive thoughts and behaviours.

Opioids: A class of pain-relieving drugs that interact with specific receptors in the nervous system.

Optic nerve: A bundle of nerve fibres that transmit visual information from the eye to the brain.

236

Oral Contraceptive Pills: Medications containing hormones to prevent pregnancy.

Oxidative stress: Imbalance between free radicals and antioxidants, linked to various diseases.

Oxygen demand: The amount of oxygen required by the body's cells.

Oxygen-carrying capacity: The ability of red blood cells to transport oxygen.

Oxygenated blood: Blood containing a high level of oxygen, usually leaving the lungs.

Oxygenated blood: Blood containing a high level of oxygen.

Pancreatitis: Inflammation of the pancreas.

Paradoxical disinhibition: A phenomenon where a medication causes an unexpected increase in specific behaviours.

Paranoid: Experiencing extreme suspicion or fear, often without rational basis.

Paranoid: Experiencing unfounded or exaggerated

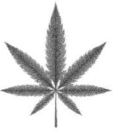

fears and suspicions.

Parkinson's disease: A neurological disorder characterized by tremors and movement difficulties.

Partial pressure gradient: Difference in partial pressures that drives the movement of gases during gaseous exchange.

Partial pressure gradient: The difference in partial pressures between two areas that drives gas exchange.

Partial pressures: The pressure exerted by a single gas within a mixture of gases.

Particulate matter: Small particles suspended in the air, often produced by combustion processes.

Particulate matter: Tiny particles suspended in the air, often emitted during combustion processes.

Pathophysiology: The study of the changes in normal physiological processes leading to disease.

Perception: The process of recognizing and interpreting sensory information from the environment.

Perception: The process of recognizing and interpreting sensory information from the environment.

Perforation: A hole or opening in a structure.

Peripheral vision: The ability to see objects and movement outside of the direct line of sight.

237

Pharmacokinetics: Study of how drugs are absorbed, distributed, metabolized, and excreted in the body.

Pharmacology: Study of drugs, their actions, interactions, and effects on the body.

Phlegm: Thick mucus produced by the respiratory system, often due to inflammation.

Phospholipids: Molecules that constitute the lipid bilayer of cell membranes, with hydrophilic heads and hydrophobic tails.

Physical dependence: Reliance on a substance to function normally.

Physiological functions: Functions and processes that occur within the body to maintain homeostasis and health.

Physiological functions: Normal bodily processes required for survival and optimal functioning.

Physiology: The study of how living organisms func-

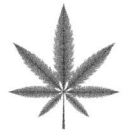

tion and interact with their environments.

Physiology: The study of the normal functions of living organisms and their parts.

Placebo effect: Improvement in symptoms due to belief in treatment rather than its inherent properties.

Placenta: An organ connecting the fetus to the uterine wall, providing nutrients and oxygen during pregnancy.

Plasticity: The brain's ability to adapt and reorganize itself in response to experiences.

Polycyclic aromatic hydrocarbons: Chemical compounds present in tobacco smoke and other environmental sources, some of which are carcinogenic.

Prefrontal cortex: The front part of the brain involved in decision-making, behaviour, and personality.

Prenatal period: The time during pregnancy before birth.

Prenatal: Relating to the period before birth.

Primary open-angle glaucoma: The most common form of glaucoma, often leading to gradual vision loss.

Product safety: Ensuring that products meet quality standards and are safe for consumer use.

Profuse sweating: Excessive sweating.

Pseudo-deficiency: A condition resembling a deficiency but caused by other factors.

Psyche: The totality of the human mind, including conscious and unconscious elements.

Psychiatry: A medical specialty focusing on the diagnosis and treatment of mental disorders.

Psychoactive compound: A substance that affects brain function, altering perception, mood, consciousness, or behaviour.

Psychoactive properties: Refers to the ability of a substance, like THC in cannabis, to affect the brain and alter mental processes, mood, perception, or behaviour.

Psychoanalysis: A therapeutic approach to treating mental health issues by exploring unconscious thoughts and emotions.

Psychological dependence: Emotional reliance on a substance.

Psychosis: A mental state where a person loses touch

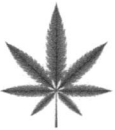

with reality, experiencing delusions, hallucinations, and impaired thinking. High doses of THC may induce temporary psychosis.

Psychotherapy: Therapeutic interventions aiming to improve mental health through talk-based methods.

Psychotic disorders: Mental health conditions characterized by impaired thinking, emotions, and perceptions. Cannabis use, particularly with high THC content, may increase the risk of psychotic disorders in vulnerable individuals.

Pulmonary gas exchange: The exchange of oxygen and carbon dioxide between the alveoli and blood in the lungs.

RBC count: The number of red blood cells in a blood sample.

Recreational users: Individuals who use substances like cannabis for enjoyment and leisure rather than medical necessity.

Recreational: Pertaining to the non-medical, leisure use of substances or activities for enjoyment.

Red blood cells: Cells responsible for carrying oxygen throughout the body.

Refractory asthma: Severe asthma that does not respond well to standard treatments.

239

Residual cannabis metabolites: Traces of cannabis components in the body after use.

Respiration: The process of inhaling oxygen and exhaling carbon dioxide to provide the body with oxygen for cellular metabolism.

Respiratory irritation: Inflammation and discomfort in the respiratory tract.

Respiratory issues: Health problems affecting the lungs and breathing, which can be exacerbated by smoking cannabis.

Respiratory system: The bodily system responsible for bringing oxygen into the body and expelling carbon dioxide.

Responsible marketing practices: Ethical and transparent approaches to promoting products that prioritize consumer well-being.

Restlessness: Inability to sit still or relax.

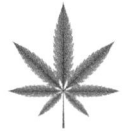

Schizophrenia: A severe mental disorder characterized by disorganized thoughts, hallucinations, and delusions.

Scientific discovery: Identification of new knowledge or insights through research and experimentation.

Scientific evidence: Data and results from rigorously conducted research studies that support or refute a hypothesis.

Scientific inquiry: Process of exploring and investigating phenomena using systematic methods to form conclusions based on evidence.

Scientific research: Systematic investigation of a topic using controlled methodologies to gain new knowledge or insights.

Sedating effects: Effects that promote relaxation and sleepiness.

Sedation: A calming effect that can lead to drowsiness and reduced alertness.

Seizures: Sudden, abnormal electrical activity in the brain that can result in various symptoms, such as convulsions or loss of consciousness.

Sensation: The process of detecting sensory stimuli, such as touch, taste, smell, sight, and hearing.

Serotonin: A neurotransmitter involved in mood regulation, appetite, and other functions.

Shortness of breath: The sensation of breathlessness or difficulty breathing.

Side effects: Unintended and often undesirable effects of a medication or treatment.

Signalling pathways: Intricate biochemical pathways that convey information within cells, regulating various cellular processes.

Slower reflexes: Delayed response to stimuli due to reduced nervous system reactivity.

Slurred speech: Impaired or difficult-to-understand speech often associated with neurological conditions.

Sodium influx: The movement of sodium ions into cells, crucial for nerve signalling.

Sperm production: The formation of sperm cells in the testes through a process called spermatogenesis.

Sperm: Male reproductive cells necessary for fertiliz-

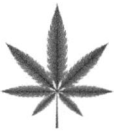

ing an egg.

Spermatogenesis: The production and development of sperm cells in the testes.

Spinal cord: A bundle of nerves running down the back that transmits signals between the brain and the body.

Sputum: Mixture of saliva and mucus coughed up from the respiratory tract.

Squamous cell carcinoma: A type of skin cancer that originates in squamous cells.

Squamous epithelial cells: Thin, flat cells that form the alveolar walls in the lungs, facilitating efficient gas exchange.

Squamous metaplasia: Transformation of cells in response to irritation, often seen in smokers.

Standard atmospheric pressure: The pressure exerted by the weight of the atmosphere at sea level, which is approximately 101.3 kilopascals (kPa) or 760 millimetres of mercury (mmHg).

Strain of cannabis: A specific variety or type of cannabis plant with distinct characteristics, including appearance, aroma, and effects.

Strain potency: The strength of a cannabis strain's effects, often influenced by its cannabinoid content.

241

Stroke: Disruption of blood supply to the brain, often leading to neurological damage.

Substance-induced psychosis: Psychotic symptoms triggered by substance use.

Sudden weakness: Rapid loss of strength in muscles.

Superego: In Freudian psychology, the part of the psyche representing moral and ethical principles.

Suppliers and manufacturers: Entities responsible for producing and distributing cannabis-related products, including medicinal cannabis.

Symptomatic relief: Alleviation of symptoms without treating the underlying cause.

Synaptic function: The process of communication between neurons at synapses.

Synaptic pruning: The elimination of unused or unnecessary synapses (connections) between neurons.

Tar: A sticky substance produced when tobacco or

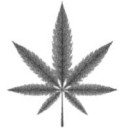

cannabis is burned, which can accumulate in the lungs.
Tar: Sticky substance produced by burning tobacco or cannabis, which can accumulate in the lungs.
Testes: Male reproductive organs responsible for producing sperm and hormones.
Testosterone: A male sex hormone responsible for various physiological processes, including the development of male reproductive tissues.
THC (Delta-9-tetrahydrocannabinol): The primary psychoactive compound in cannabis responsible for the "high" sensation and various effects on the brain and body.
THC-COOH: A metabolite of THC that can be detected in drug tests.
Therapeutic alliance: Collaborative relationship between a patient and healthcare provider.
Therapeutic index: The range between the dose of a medication that produces therapeutic effects and the dose that causes adverse effects.
Therapeutic: Relating to the treatment or management of a medical condition to restore health or alleviate symptoms.
Tolerance: The reduced effectiveness of a substance with repeated use, requiring higher doses to achieve the same effects.
Trabecular meshwork: A network of tissue that drains fluid from the eye, regulating intraocular pressure.
Trachea: The windpipe, a tube that connects the throat to the bronchi, allowing air to enter and exit the lungs.
Tremors: Involuntary shaking of body parts.
Vagina: The muscular tube connecting the uterus to the outside of the body.
Vaporizers: Devices used to heat cannabis or other substances to a temperature that produces vapour for inhalation, reducing the harmful effects associated with combustion.
Vitamin C: A water-soluble vitamin with antioxidant properties, essential for immune function and collagen synthesis.

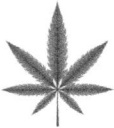

Vitamins: Essential nutrients required in small amounts for various bodily functions.
Warfarin: An anticoagulant medication to prevent blood clots.
Water-soluble: Capable of dissolving in water.
Weakness: Lack of physical strength or energy.
Wheezing: High-pitched sound during breathing caused by narrowed airways.
Wheezing: High-pitched whistling sound produced during breathing, often indicating narrowed airways.
Withdrawal symptoms: Physical and psychological effects experienced when discontinuing a substance.

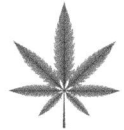

For Further Reading:

1. Abarikwu SO, Akiri OF, Durojaiye MA, Adenike A. Combined administration of delta-9-tetrahy drocannabinol (THC) and methyl mercury (MeHg) alters testosterone level and histopathology of testes in male mice. Eur J Med Res. 2008;13(10): 468-472. doi:10.1186/2047-783x-13-10-468
2. Abbott, C. W., & Nakamura, L. Y. (2021). The Fetal Alcohol Syndrome: A Literature Review. Journal of Prenatal Medicine, 15(1), 1-9.
3. Abrams, D. I. (2018). The therapeutic effects of Cannabis and cannabinoids: An update from the National Academies of Sciences, Engineering and Medicine report. European journal of internal medicine, 49, 7-11.
4. Abrams, D. I. (2018). The therapeutic effects of Cannabis and cannabinoids: An update from the National Academies of Sciences, Engineering and Medicine report. European journal of internal medicine, 49, 7-11.
5. Aggarwal SK. Cannabinergic Pain Medicine: A Concise Clinical Primer and Survey of Randomized-controlled Trial Results. Clinical Journal of Pain. 2013 Jul;29(7):649-59.
6. Agrawal, A., et al. (2012). The association between cannabis involvement and suicidal thoughts and behaviours: A longitudinal study of young adults. JAMA Psychiatry, 69(9), 901-907.
7. Alberts, B., Johnson, A., Lewis, J., Raff, M., Roberts, K., & Walter, P. (2002). Molecular Biology of the Cell (4th ed.). Garland Science.
8. Alberts, B., Johnson, A., Lewis, J., Raff, M., Roberts, K., Walter, P. (2014). Molecular Biology of the Cell (6th ed.). Garland Science.

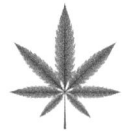

245

9. Amato, L., Davoli, M., Minozzi, S., Ferroni, E., Ali, R., & Ferri, M. (2011). Methadone at tapered doses for the management of opioid withdrawal. Cochrane Database of Systematic Reviews, 2011(2), CD003409.

10. American Academy of Family Physicians. (2017). Self-care and over-the-counter products. Retrieved from https://www.aafp.org/afp/2017/0801/p177.html

11. American Academy of Ophthalmology. (2021). Glaucoma. Retrieved from https://www.aao.org/eye-health/diseases/glaucoma

12. American Academy of Ophthalmology. (2021). Marijuana and Eye Health: What You Need to Know. Retrieved from https://www.aao.org/eye-health/tips-prevention/marijuana-eye-health

13. American Cancer Society. (2021). Non-Small Cell Lung Cancer. Retrieved from https://www.cancer.org/cancer/lung-cancer/about/what-is.html

14. American Cancer Society. (2021). Signs and Symptoms of Brain and Spinal Cord Tumors in Adults. Retrieved from https://www.cancer.org/cancer/brain-spinal-cord-tumors-adults/detection-diagnosis-staging/signs-symptoms.html

15. American Cancer Society. (2021). What Causes Lung Cancer? Retrieved from https://www.cancer.org/cancer/lung-cancer/causes-risks-prevention/what-causes.html

16. American College of Obstetricians and Gynecologists. (2013). Nutrition during pregnancy. Retrieved from https://www.acog.org/womens-health/faqs/nutrition-during-pregnancy

17. American College of Obstetricians and Gynecologists. (2019). Committee Opinion No. 743: Low-Dose Aspirin Use During

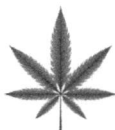

Pregnancy. Obstetrics and Gynecology, 133(1), e44-e52.

18. American College of Obstetricians and Gynecologists. (2020). Committee Opinion No. 711: Opioid Use and Opioid Use Disorder in Pregnancy. Obstetrics and Gynecology, 135(4), e210-e220.

19. American College of Obstetricians and Gynecologists. (2020). Committee Opinion No. 767: Alcohol use in pregnancy. Obstetrics & Gynecology, 135(2), e72-e80.

20. American Diabetes Association. (2022). Standards of Medical Care in Diabetes - 2022. Diabetes Care, 45(Supplement 1), S3-S234.

21. American Heart Association. (2018). Homocysteine, folic acid, and cardiovascular disease. Retrieved from https://www.heart.org/en/health-topics/consumer-healthcare/what-is-cardiovascular-disease/homocysteine-folic-acid-and-cardiovascular-disease

22. American Heart Association. (2020). Homocysteine and MTHFR Mutations: What's the Connection? Retrieved from https://www.heart.org/en/health-topics/consumer-healthcare/what-is-cardiovascular-disease/homocysteine-and-mthfr-mutations-whats-the-connection

23. American Heart Association. (2020). Smoking and cardiovascular disease. Retrieved from https://www.heart.org/en/healthy-living/healthy-lifestyle/quit-smoking-tobacco/smoking-and-cardiovascular-disease

24. American Heart Association. (2020). Warning Signs of a Heart Attack. Retrieved from https://www.heart.org/en/health-topics/heart-attack/warning-signs-of-a-heart-attack

25. American Heart Association. (2021). Heart Attack Symptoms in Women.

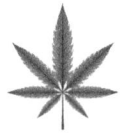

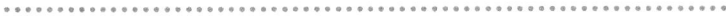

247

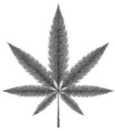

Retrieved from https://www.heart.org/en/
health-topics/heart-attack/warning-signs-of-a-
heart-attack/heart-attack-symptoms-in-women

26. American Lung Association. (2021).
Learn About Lung Cancer. Retrieved from
https://www.lung.org/lung-health-diseases/
lung-disease-lookup/lung-cancer/learn-about-
lung-cancer

27. American Medical Association. (2021).
Opinion 2.1.1 - The Principles of Medical
Ethics. Retrieved from https://www.ama-assn.
org/delivering-care/ethics/principles-
medical-ethics

28. American Pharmacists Association. (2021).
Self-care and nonprescription pharmacother
apy. Retrieved from
https://www.pharmacist.com/sites/
default/files/files/MTM%20Central/
MTM-Chapter12-Self-Care-and-
Nonprescription-Pharmacotherapy.pdf

29. American Psychiatric Association. (2013).
Diagnostic and statistical manual of mental
disorders (5th ed.). Arlington, VA:
American Psychiatric Publishing.

30. American Psychiatric Association. (2013).
Diagnostic and Statistical Manual of Mental
Disorders (5th ed.). Washington, DC: American
Psychiatric Publishing.

31. American Statistical Association. (2016).
ASA statement on statistical significance
and p-values. Retrieved from
https://www.amstat.org/asa/files/pdfs/
P-ValueStatement.pdf

32. American Stroke Association. (2021).
Stroke Warning Signs and Symptoms.
Retrieved from https://www.stroke.org/en/
about-stroke/stroke-warning-signs-and-symptoms

33. Aryana, A., & Williams, M. A. (2007).
Marijuana as a trigger of cardiovascular events:
speculation or scientific certainty?
International Journal of Cardiology, 118(2), 141-144.

34. Atalay S, Jarocka-Karpowicz I, Skrzydlewska E. Antioxidative and Anti-Inflammatory Properties of Cannabidiol. Antioxidants (Basel). 2019;9(1):21. doi:10.3390/antiox9010021

35. Atwood BK, Mackie K. CB2: a cannabinoid receptor with an identity crisis. Br J Pharmacol. 2010;160(3):467-479. doi:10.1111/j.1476-5381.2010.00729.x

36. Back, D. J., Orme, M. L. E., & Breckenridge, A. M. (1982). Pharmacokinetic drug interactions between oral contraceptive steroids and drugs used to treat epilepsy. Clinical Pharmacokinetics, 7(6), 533-552.

37. Baio, J., Wiggins, L., Christensen, D. L., Maenner, M. J., Daniels, J., Warren, Z., ... & Dowling, N. F. (2018). Prevalence of autism spectrum disorder among children aged 8 years—Autism and Developmental Disabilities Monitoring Network, 11 sites, United States, 2014. MMWR. Surveillance Summaries, 67(6), 1-23.

38. Batalla A, et al. The impact of cannabis use on cognitive functioning in adolescents and young adults: A systematic review. Addiction. 2013;108(3):417-425.

39. Batalla, A., Bhattacharyya, S., Yücel, M., Fusar-Poli, P., Crippa, J. A., Nogué, S., ... & Martin-Santos, R. (2013). Structural and functional imaging studies in chronic cannabis users: a systematic review of adolescent and adult findings. PloS One, 8(2), e55821.

40. Battistella, G., Fornari, E., Annoni, J. M., Chtioui, H., Dao, K., Fabritius, M., ... & Giroud, C. (2014). Long-term effects of cannabis on brain structure. Neuropsychopharmacology, 39(9), 2041-2048.

41. Beauchamp, T. L., & Childress, J. F. (2019). Principles of biomedical ethics. Oxford University Press.

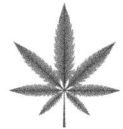

249

42. Benowitz, N. L. (2010). Nicotine addiction. New England Journal of Medicine, 362(24), 2295-2303.
43. Bertino Jr, J. S. (1995). Erythromycin, clarithromycin, and azithromycin: are the differences real? Clinical Therapeutics, 17(5), 913-933.
44. Bhattacharyya, S., Egerton, A., Kim, E., Rosso, L., Riano Barros, D., Hammers, A., ... & McGuire, P. (2017). Acute induction of anxiety in humans by delta-9-tetrahydrocannabinol related to amygdalar cannabinoid-1 (CB1) receptors. Scientific Reports, 7(1), 1-11.
45. Bhattacharyya, S., Morrison, P. D., Fusar-Poli, P., et al. (2010). Opposite effects of delta-9-tetrahydrocannabinol and cannabidiol on human brain function and psychopathology. Neuropsychopharmacology, 35(3), 764-774.
46. Blaak, E. E., Antoine, J. M., Benton, D., Björck, I., Bozzetto, L., Brouns, F., ... & Vinoy, S. (2012). Impact of postprandial glycaemia on health and prevention of disease. Obesity Reviews, 13(10), 923-984.
47. Blease, C., Bernstein, M. H., & Gaab, J. (2017). Intuition and evidence—uneasy bedfellows? The BMJ Opinion. Retrieved from https://blogs.bmj.com/bmj/2017/07/14/charles-blease-et-al-intuition-and-evidence-uneasy-bedfellows/
48. Blessing EM, Steenkamp MM, Manzanares J, et al. Cannabidiol as a Potential Treatment for Anxiety Disorders. Neurotherapeutics. 2015 Oct;12(4):825-36.
49. Boehnke, K. F., & Wayne, P. M. (2017). Cannabinoids in the management of chronic pain: a novel therapeutic approach. The Yale Journal of Biology and Medicine, 90(3), 403-411.
50. Bonaccorso, S., & Pariante, C. M. (2019). Is

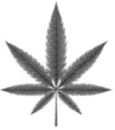

250

There a Role for Personalised Medicine in the Treatment of Mood Disorders? The Role of Pharmacogenomics in Antidepressant Therapy. The Psychiatric Clinics of North America, 42(1), 71-87.

51. Bonn-Miller MO, Loflin MJE, Thomas BF, Marcu JP, Hyke T, Vandrey R. Labeling Accuracy of Cannabidiol Extracts Sold Online. JAMA. 2017;318(17):1708-1709. doi:10.1001/jama.2017.11909

52. Bonnet, U., & Preuss, U. W. (2017). The cannabis withdrawal syndrome: current insights. Substance Abuse and Rehabilitation, 8, 9-37.

53. Bordin, E. S. (1979). The generalizability of the psychoanalytic concept of the working alliance. Psychotherapy: Theory, Research & Practice, 16(3), 252-260.

54. Brunton LL, Hilal-Dandan R, Knollmann BC. Goodman & Gilman's The Pharmacological Basis of Therapeutics. 13th edition. McGraw-Hill Education; 2017.

55. Budney, A. J., & Borodovsky, J. T. (2017). The potential impact of cannabis legalization on the development of cannabis use disorders. Preventive Medicine, 104, 31-36.

56. Budney, A. J., Hughes, J. R., Moore, B. A., & Vandrey, R. (2004). Review of the validity and significance of cannabis withdrawal syndrome. American Journal of Psychiatry, 161(11), 1967-1977.

57. Budney, A. J., Roffman, R., Stephens, R. S., & Walker, D. (2007). Marijuana dependence and its treatment. Addiction Science & Clinical Practice, 4(1), 4-16.

58. Bybee, R. W. (1997). Achieving scientific literacy: From purposes to practices. Heinemann.

59. Campbell, N. A., et al. (2019). Biology: Concepts and Connections (9th ed.). Pearson.

60. Caulkins, J. P., Kilmer, B., & Kleiman, M. A.

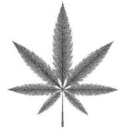

251

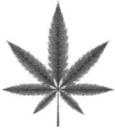

(2016). Marijuana legalization: What everyone needs to know. Oxford University Press.

61. Cenkowski, M., & O'Reilly, R. A. (1990). Differential interaction of erythromycin and clarithromycin with warfarin in patients. Clinical Pharmacology & Therapeutics, 48(3), 305-314.

62. Centers for Disease Control and Prevention. (2020). Risk Factors for Lung Cancer. Retrieved from https://www.cdc.gov/cancer/lung/basic_info/risk_factors.htm

63. Centers for Disease Control and Prevention. (2020). Smoking During Pregnancy. Retrieved from https://www.cdc.gov/tobacco/basic_information/pregnancy/index.htm

64. Centers for Disease Control and Prevention. (2021). Alcohol and Pregnancy. Retrieved from https://www.cdc.gov/ncbddd/spanish/fasd/alcohol-use.html

65. Centers for Disease Control and Prevention. (2021). Fetal Alcohol Spectrum Disorders (FASDs): Data and Statistics. Retrieved from https://www.cdc.gov/ncbddd/fasd/data.html

66. Centers for Disease Control and Prevention. (2021). HIV/AIDS: Basic Information. Retrieved from https://www.cdc.gov/hiv/basics/index.html

67. Centers for Disease Control and Prevention. (2021). Pregnancy and alcohol. Retrieved from https://www.cdc.gov/ncbddd/spanish/fasd/facts.html

68. Centers for Disease Control and Prevention. (2021). Smoking and pregnancy. Retrieved from https://www.cdc.gov/tobacco/basic_information/health_effects/pregnancy/index.htm

69. Chandra, S., Lata, H., ElSohly, M. A., & Walker, L. A. (Eds.). (2017). Cannabis sativa L.-Botany and Biotechnology. Springer.

70. Chen, C. Y., O'Brien, B. C., & Anthony, J. C. (2005). Who becomes cannabis dependent

soon after onset of use? Epidemiological evidence from the United States: 2000-2001. Drug and Alcohol Dependence, 79(1), 11-22.

71. Cole, B. F., Baron, J. A., Sandler, R. S., Haile, R. W., Ahnen, D. J., Bresalier, R. S., ... & Burke, C. A. (2007). Folic acid for the prevention of colorectal adenomas: a randomized clinical trial. JAMA, 297(21), 2351-2359.

72. Colizzi, M., McGuire, P., Pertwee, R. G., & Bhattacharyya, S. (2016). Effect of cannabis on glutamate signalling in the brain: A systematic review of human and animal evidence. Neuroscience and Biobehavioral Reviews, 64, 359-381.

73. Conner, S. N., Bedell, V., Lipsey, K., Macones, G. A., Cahill, A. G., Tuuli, M. G. (2016). Maternal marijuana use and neonatal morbidity. American Journal of Obstetrics and Gynecology, 215(4), 506.e1-506.e7.

74. Cooper, Z. D., & Haney, M. (2009). Cannabis reinforcement and dependence: role of the cannabinoid CB1 receptor. Addiction Biology, 14(3), 289-300.

75. Corsi, D. J., Walsh, L., Weiss, D., & Hsu, H. (2020). Association Between Self-reported Prenatal Cannabis Use and Maternal, Perinatal, and Neonatal Outcomes. JAMA: Journal of the American Medical Association, 324(6), 592-604. doi:10.1001/jama.2020.14421

76. Cotran, R. S., Kumar, V., Collins, T., & Robbins, S. L. (1999). Robbins Pathologic Basis of Disease (6th ed.). W. B. Saunders Company.

77. Crean, R. D., Crane, N. A., & Mason, B. J. (2011). An evidence-based review of acute and long-term effects of cannabis use on executive cognitive functions. Journal of Addiction Medicine, 5(1), 1-8.

78. Curtis, A. B. (2017). Approach to the adult patient with anemia. In Goldman-Cecil Medicine (26th ed., pp. 319-325). Elsevier.

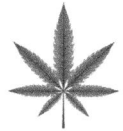

79. Czeizel, A. E., & Dudás, I. (1992). Prevention of the first occurrence of neural-tube defects by periconceptional vitamin supplementation. New England Journal of Medicine, 327(26), 1832-1835.

80. Daly, A. K. (2006). Pharmacogenetics: The role of inherited genetic differences in drug disposition and response. Clinical Pharmacology & Therapeutics, 79(5), 472-485.

81. Dantzker, D. R. (2011). The pathophysiology of respiratory failure. In Principles of critical care (pp. 461-473). McGraw-Hill Education.

82. Dartt, D. A. (2013). Neural regulation of lacrimal gland secretory processes: Relevance in dry eye diseases. Progress in Retinal and Eye Research, 45, 168-176.

83. Davies, M., & Hayes, J. (2019). Interpreting the drug–drug interaction between warfarin and flucloxacillin. British Journal of Clinical Pharmacology, 85(1), 208-211.

84. De Sousa Fernandes Perna, E. B., Moreno, A., & Gil, F. (2018). Alcohol-Drug Interactions. Journal of Clinical Medicine, 7(10), 332.

85. Devinsky O, Cross JH, Laux L, et al. Trial of Cannabidiol for Drug-Resistant Seizures in the Dravet Syndrome. N Engl J Med. 2017;376(21):2011-2020. doi:10.1056/NEJMoa1611618

86. Di Forti M, Quattrone D, Freeman TP, et al. The contribution of cannabis use to variation in the incidence of psychotic disorder across Europe (EU-GEI): a multicentre case-control study. Lancet Psychiatry. 2019 Mar;6(5):427-36.

87. Di Forti, M., Marconi, A., Carra, E., Fraietta, S., Trotta, A., Bonomo, M., ... & Murray, R. M. (2015). Proportion of patients in south London with first-episode psychosis attributable to use of high potency cannabis: a case-control study.

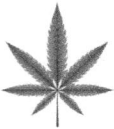

The Lancet Psychiatry, 2(3), 233-238.
88. Di Forti, M., Quattrone, D., Freeman, T. P., Tripoli, G., Gayer-Anderson, C., Quigley, H., ... & Ferraro, L. (2019). The contribution of cannabis use to variation in the incidence of psychotic disorder across Europe (EU-GEI): a multicentre case-control study. The Lancet Psychiatry, 6(5), 427-436.
89. Di Forti, M., Quattrone, D., Freeman, T. P., Tripoli, G., Gayer-Anderson, C., Quigley, H., ... & Rodriguez, V. (2019). The contribution of cannabis use to variation in the incidence of psychotic disorder across Europe (EU-GEI): a multicentre case-control study. The Lancet Psychiatry, 6(5), 427-436.
90. Dinesen, B., Nonnemann, M., Lindeman, D., Toft, E., Kidholm, K., & Jethwani, K. (2019). Personalized Telehealth in the Future: A Global Research Agenda. Journal of Medical Internet Research, 21(4), e12831.
91. Dougherty, T. G. (2015). Microcytic anemia. New England Journal of Medicine, 372(19), 1832-1843.
92. Earleywine, M. (2002). Understanding Marijuana: A New Look at the Scientific Evidence. Oxford University Press.
93. Emanuel, E. J., & Dubler, N. N. (1995). Preserving the physician-patient relationship in the era of managed care. Jama, 273(4), 323-329.
94. EMCDDA. (2021). Perspectives on Drugs: Drug Consumption Rooms: An Overview of Provision and Evidence. Retrieved from https://www.emcdda.europa.eu/publications/pods/drug-consumption-rooms_en
95. Ernst, E. (2008). Complementary and alternative medicine: What is it all about? Occupational and Environmental Medicine, 65(11), 759-766.
96. Ernst, E., & Schmidt, K. (2004). Alternative medicine-A critical assessment of 150

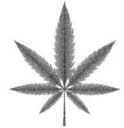

modalities. Springer.

97. Fergusson, D. M., Lynskey, M. T., & Horwood, L. J. (1996). Childhood exposure to cannabis and psychotic symptoms in adolescence and early adulthood. Psychological Medicine, 26(4), 801-811.

98. FoodData Central. (n.d.). U.S. Department of Agriculture. Retrieved from https://fdc.nal. usda.gov/

99. Frisancho, A. R. (2017). High-altitude adaptation: Unique challenges in water balance. In Human Adaptation to Extreme Stress (2nd ed., pp. 225-236). Routledge.

100. Ghasemiesfe, M., Ravi, D., Vali, M., Korenstein, D., & Keyhani, S. (2018). Marijuana use, respiratory symptoms, and pulmonary function: A systematic review and meta-analysis. Annals of Internal Medicine, 169(2), 106-115.

101. Giusti, R. M., Iwamoto, K., Hatch, E. E., & Titus-Ernstoff, L. (1995). DES Exposure and the Risk of Breast Cancer. Cancer Causes & Control, 6(1), 75-82.

102. Glover, V. (2015). Prenatal stress and its effects on the fetus and the child: Possible underlying biological mechanisms. In Handbook of Developmental Psychopathology (2nd ed.). Springer.

103. Goodman, S. N., Fanelli, D., & Ioannidis, J. P. (2016). What does research reproducibility mean? Science Translational Medicine, 8(341), 341ps12.

104. Government of Canada. (2021). Information for health care professionals: Cannabis (marihuana, marijuana) and the cannabinoids. Retrieved from https://www.canada.ca/en/health-canada/ services/drugs-medication/cannabis/ information-medical-practitioners/ information-health-care-professionals- cannabis-cannabinoids.html

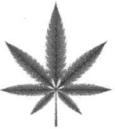

105. Goyal, S., Chauhan, S. K., & Dana, R. (2019). Blockade of prolymphangiogenic vascular endothelial growth factor C in dry eye disease. Archives of Ophthalmology, 137(9), 992-994.
106. Grady, C. (2017). Enduring and emerging challenges of informed consent. New England Journal of Medicine, 376(9), 856-863.
107. Green, E. C. (2001). The role of belief in integrative medicine. Alternative Therapies in Health and Medicine, 7(2), 18-19.
108. Greenfield, G., Foley, K., Majeed, A., & Raftery, J. (2016). Young people's clinic use and associations with clinical outcomes: population-based study in primary care. British Journal of General Practice, 66(652), e591-e597.
109. Greenland, S., Pearl, J., & Robins, J. M. (1999). Causal diagrams for epidemiologic research. Epidemiology, 10(1), 37-48.
110. Grinspoon, P. (2020). Medical Marijuana and the Eye. Harvard Health Publishing. Retrieved from https://www.health.harvard.edu/blog/medical-marijuana-and-the-eye-2019010915746
111. Grotenhermen, F., & Russo, E. (Eds.). (2002). Cannabis and cannabinoids: Pharmacology, toxicology, and therapeutic potential. Haworth Press.
112. Gunn, J. K., Rosales, C. B., Center, K. E., Nuñez, A. V., Gibson, S. J., Christ, C., ... & Georgieff, M. K. (2016). Prenatal exposure to cannabis and maternal and child health outcomes: a systematic review and meta-analysis. BMJ Open, 6(4), e009986.
113. Gunnar, M. R., & Quevedo, K. M. (2007). Early care experiences and HPA axis regulation in children: A mechanism for later trauma vulnerability. Progress in Brain Research, 167, 137-149.
114. Hackam, D. G., & Anand, S. S. (2003). Emerging risk factors for atherosclerotic

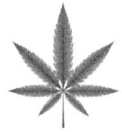

257

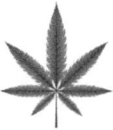

vascular disease: a critical review of the evidence. JAMA, 290(7), 932-940.

115. Hall W, Degenhardt L. Adverse health effects of non-medical cannabis use. Lancet. 2009 Oct 17;374(9698):1383-91.

116. Hall, J. E. (2015). Guyton and Hall textbook of medical physiology (13th ed.). Elsevier.

117. Hall, M. A., Zheng, B., Dugan, E., Camacho, F., Kidd, K. E., Mishra, A. K., ... & Trust Investigators. (2001). Measuring patients' trust in their primary care providers. Medical Care Research and Review, 58(3), 330-349.

118. Hall, W., & Degenhardt, L. (2009). Adverse health effects of non-medical cannabis use. The Lancet, 374(9698), 1383-1391.

119. Hall, W., & Degenhardt, L. (2020). Adverse health effects of non-medical cannabis use. The Lancet, 395(10213), 1176-1188.

120. Hall, W., & Degenhardt, L. (2020). Adverse health effects of non-medical cannabis use. The Lancet, 395(10235), 1740-1742.

121. Harm Reduction International. (2021). What is Harm Reduction? Retrieved from https://www.hri.global/what-is-harm-reduction

122. Hartman, R. L., Brown, T. L., Milavetz, G., Spurgin, A., Gorelick, D. A., & Gaffney, G. (2016). Controlled cannabis vaporizer administration: Blood and plasma cannabinoids with and without alcohol. Clinical Chemistry, 62(12), 1572-1581.

123. Hartman, R. L., Huestis, M. A. (2013). Cannabis effects on driving skills. Clinical Chemistry, 59(3), 478-492.

124. Harvard Health Publishing. (2018). Medical Marijuana. Retrieved from https://www.health.harvard.edu/blog/medical-marijuana-2018011513085

125. Harvard Health Publishing. (2019). What to do when depression doesn't go away.

258

Retrieved from https://www.health.harvard.edu/mind-and-mood/what_to_do_when_depression_doesnt_go_away

126. Harvard Health Publishing. (2021). What are the real risks of antidepressants? Retrieved from https://www.health.harvard.edu/mind-and-mood/what-are-the-real-risks-of-antidepressants

127. Hasin DS, et al. Prevalence of Marijuana Use Disorders in the United States Between 2001-2002 and 2012-2013. JAMA Psychiatry. 2015;72(12):1235-1242. doi:10.1001/jamapsychiatry.2015.1858

128. Hazekamp, A., & Grotenhermen, F. (2010). Re view on clinical studies with cannabis and cannabinoids 2005-2009. Cannabinoids, 5(1), 1-21.

129. Hensley, A. N., & DeVilbiss, E. A. (2019). The impact of prenatal and perinatal exposures on autism: a systematic review. Autism Research, 12(2), 184-203.

130. Herbst, A. L., & Poskanzer, D. C. (1974). Adenocarcinoma of the Vagina. New England Journal of Medicine, 290(9), 431-432.

131. Hergenrather, J. Y., Capler, R., & De Jong, M. (2017). Cannabis use patterns and motives: A comparison of younger, middle-aged, and older medical cannabis dispensary patients. Cannabis and Cannabinoid Research, 2(1), 144-151.

132. Hernán, M. A., & Robins, J. M. (2020). Causal inference: What if. CRC Press.

133. Hesse, L. M., von Moltke, L. L., & Greenblatt, D. J. (2007). Clinically important drug interactions with zopiclone, zolpidem and zaleplon. CNS Drugs, 21(3), 191-206.

134. Hill KP. Medical Marijuana for Treatment of Chronic Pain and Other Medical and Psychiatric Problems: A Clinical Review. JAMA. 2015;313(24):2474-2483. doi:10.1001/jama.2015.6199

135. Hill, A. J. (2007). The psychology of food craving. Proceedings of the Nutrition Society,

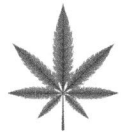

259

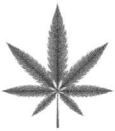

66(2), 277-285.

136. Hill, K. P. (2015). Medical marijuana for treatment of chronic pain and other medical and psychiatric problems: A clinical review. JAMA, 313(24), 2474-2483.

137. Hindocha C, Freeman TP, Schafer G, et al. Acute effects of cannabinoids on memory in humans: a review. Psychopharmacology (Berl). 2017;234(8):1121-1134. doi:10.1007/s00213-017-4756-9

138. Holbrook, A. M., Pereira, J. A., Labiris, R., McDonald, H., & Douketis, J. D. (2005). Systematic overview of warfarin and its drug and food interactions. Archives of Internal Medicine, 165(10), 1095-1106.

139. Horscroft, J. A., & Murray, A. J. (2017). Skeletal muscle metabolism in health and disease: A role for hypoxia. Experimental Physiology, 102(11), 1357-1372. doi: 10.1113/EP086287

140. Horvath, A. O., & Bedi, R. P. (2002). The alliance. Psychotherapy, 38(4), 365-372.

141. Huestis MA. Human cannabinoid pharmacokinetics. Chem Biodivers. 2007;4(8):1770-1804. doi:10.1002/cbdv.200790152

142. Huestis, M. A. (2007). Human cannabinoid pharmacokinetics. Chemistry & Biodiversity, 4(8), 1770-1804.

143. Huestis, M. A. (2009). Pharmacokinetics and metabolism of the plant cannabinoids, Δ9-tetrahydrocannabinol, cannabidiol and cannabinol. Handb Exp Pharmacol, 168, 657-690.

144. Huestis, M. A., Mitchell, J. M., & Cone, E. J. (1996). Urinary excretion profiles of 11-nor-9-carboxy-Δ9-tetrahydrocannabinol in humans after single smoked doses of marijuana. Journal of Analytical Toxicology, 20(6), 441-452.

145. Hug, C. C., Murphy, M. R., & Roe, D. A. (1984).

The effect of enzyme induction on thiopental and pancuronium anesthesia and their recovery in rabbits. Anesthesiology, 60(1), 37-42.

146. Hujoel, P. P. (2016). Causal reasoning in dental research. Journal of Dental Research, 95(5), 485-486.

147. Hunninghake, R. (1999). Lung Antioxidant Defense. Proceedings of the American Thoracic Society, 16(2), 139-143.

148. Hurd, Y. L., Yoon, M., Manini, A. F., Hernandez, S., Olmedo, R., Ostman, M., & Jutras-Aswad, D. (2015). Early phase in the development of cannabidiol as a treatment for addiction: opioid relapse takes initial center stage. Neurotherapeutics, 12(4), 807-815.

149. Hurd, Y. L., Yoon, M., Manini, A. F., Hernandez, S., Olmedo, R., Ostman, M., & Jutras-Aswad, D. (2015). Early Phase in the Development of Cannabidiol as a Treatment for Addiction: Opioid Relapse Takes Initial Center Stage. Neurotherapeutics, 12(4), 807-815. doi: 10.1007/s13311-015-0373-7

150. Insel, T. R., & Quirion, R. (2005). Psychiatric disorders as disorders of brain circuits. Neuroscience, 6, 121-131.

151. Ioannidis, J. P. (2005). Why most published research findings are false. PLoS Medicine, 2(8), e124.

152. Jampel, H. D. (2020). The Potential Role of Cannabinoids in Glaucoma. Survey of Ophthalmology, 65(5), 521-527.

153. Jatoi, A., Windschitl, H. E., Loprinzi, C. L., Sloan, J. A., Dakhil, S. R., Mailliard, J. A., ... & Fitch, T. R. (2002). Dronabinol versus megestrol acetate versus combination therapy for cancer-associated anorexia: A North Central Cancer Treatment Group study. Journal of Clinical Oncology, 20(2), 567-573.

154. Jensen, M. D., Ryan, D. H., Apovian, C. M., Ard, J. D., Comuzzie, A. G., Donato, K. A.,

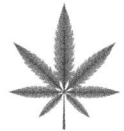

... & Yanovski, S. Z. (2014). 2013 AHA/ACC/TOS guideline for the management of overweight and obesity in adults: a report of the American College of Cardiology/American Heart Association Task Force on Practice Guidelines and The Obesity Society. Journal of the American College of Cardiology, 63(25 Part B), 2985-3023.

155. Johnson, S. B., Park, H. S., Gross, C. P., & Yu, J. B. (2018). Complementary medicine, refusal of conventional cancer therapy, and survival among patients with curable cancers. JAMA Oncology, 4(10), 1375-1381.

156. Jouanjus, É., Lapeyre-Mestre, M., & Micallef, J. (2014). Cannabis use: Signal of increasing risk of serious cardiovascular disorders. Journal of the American Heart Association, 3(2), e000638.

157. Juliano, L. M., & Griffiths, R. R. (2004). A critical review of caffeine withdrawal: Empirical validation of symptoms and signs, incidence, severity, and associated features. Psychopharmacology, 176(1), 1-29.

158. Kandel, E. R., Schwartz, J. H., & Jessell, T. M. (2012). Principles of Neural Science. McGraw-Hill.

159. Kando, J. C. (1987). Alcohol and oral contraceptive steroids: A review. Contraception, 36(1), 1-35.

160. Kaptchuk, T. J. (2008). Powerful placebo: the dark side of the randomized controlled trial. The Lancet, 371(9604), 1729-1730.

161. Karschner, E. L., Schwilke, E. W., Lowe, R. H., Darwin, W. D., Pope Jr, H. G., Herning, R., ... & Huestis, M. A. (2009). Implications of plasma Δ9-tetrahydrocannabinol, 11-hydroxy-Δ9-tetrahydrocannabinol, and 11-nor-9-carboxy-Δ9-tetrahydrocannabinol concentrations in chronic cannabis smokers. Journal of analytical toxicology, 33(8), 469-477.

162. Kasman AM, Thoma ME, McLain AC, Eisenberg ML. Association between use of marijuana

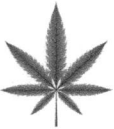

and male reproductive health:
A systematic review and meta-analysis. JAMA
Netw Open. 2019;2(11):e1916318. doi:10.1001/
jamanetworkopen.2019.16318

163. Kasper, D. L., Fauci, A. S., Hauser, S. L., Longo,
D. L., Jameson, J. L., & Loscalzo, J. (Eds.). (2015).
Harrison's Principles of Internal Medicine
(19th ed.). McGraw Hill Professional.

164. Katzung BG, Trevor AJ. Basic and Clinical
Pharmacology. 14th edition. McGraw-Hill
Education; 2018.

165. Katzung BG, Trevor AJ. Basic and Clinical
Pharmacology. 14th edition. McGraw-Hill
Education; 2018.

166. Katzung, B. G., & Trevor, A. J. (2021).
Basic & Clinical Pharmacology (16th ed.).
McGraw-Hill Education.

167. Kjeldskov, J., & Skov, M. B. (2014).
The role of anecdotes in storytelling for
motivation of computer users.
International Journal of Human-Computer
Studies, 72(2), 173-189.
doi: 10.1016/j.ijhcs.2013.10.005

168. Kooyman, G. L. (2002). Diverse divers:
physiology and behavior. Springer Science
& Business Media.

169. Kosten, T. R., & O'Connor, P. G. (2003).
Management of drug and alcohol withdrawal.
New England Journal of Medicine, 348(18),
1786-1795.

170. Kuhns, L. (2019). Cannabis and Public Health:
The Need for a Strong Evidence Base. Journal
of Adolescent Health, 65(2), 171-172.

171. Kumar, P., & Clark, M. (2012). Clinical Medicine
(8th ed.). Elsevier Health Sciences.

172. Kumar, V., Abbas, A. K., Aster, J. C., & Robbins,
S. L. (2014). Robbins basic pathology (9th ed.).
Elsevier Saunders.

173. Kwa M, Bolla KI. The potential use of
cannabinoids in erectile dysfunction and
lower urinary tract symptoms. Transl Androl

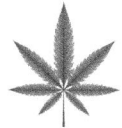

263

Urol. 2016;5(3):308-312.
doi:10.21037/tau.2016.04.04
174. Lea, M. A., & Chambers, S. (2017). Alcohol and Cancer: A Shared Pathogenesis Through Immune System Dysfunction. Seminars in Oncology Nursing, 33(3), 270–276.
175. Leach, J., & Scoones, I. (2013). The slow race: Making technology work for the poor. Demos.
176. Légaré, F., Ratté, S., Gravel, K., & Graham, I. D. (2008). Barriers and facilitators to implementing shared decision-making in clinical practice: a systematic review of health professionals' perceptions. Implementation Science, 3(1), 46.
177. Leigland, S., Schulz, K. M., & Hasan, K. M. (2013). Evolution of the Blood-Brain Barrier: A Perspective on the Discordant Timing of Gliogenesis in the Mesencephalon. Journal of Neuropathology and Experimental Neurology, 72(7), 648-654.
178. Lenné, M. G., Dietze, P. M., Triggs, T. J., Walmsley, S., Murphy, B., Redman, J. R., ... & Ng, J. F. (2010). The effects of cannabis and alcohol on simulated arterial driving: Influences of driving experience and task demand. Accident Analysis & Prevention, 42(3), 859-866.
179. Liang, W., Chikritzhs, T., & Pascal, R. (2017). Alcohol metabolism and ethnic differences. Alcohol and Alcoholism, 52(6), 628-636.
180. Lopez-Quintero C, et al. Probability and predictors of transition from first use to dependence on nicotine, alcohol, cannabis, and cocaine: results of the National Epidemiologic Survey on Alcohol and Related Conditions (NESARC). Drug Alcohol Depend. 2011;115(1-2):120-130. doi:10.1016/j.drugalcdep.2010.11.004
181. Lopez-Quintero, C., Perez de los Cobos, J., Hasin, D. S., Okuda, M., Wang, S., Grant, B. F., & Blanco, C. (2011). Probability and predictors

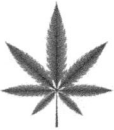

264

of transition from first use to dependence on nicotine, alcohol, cannabis, and cocaine: results of the National Epidemiologic Survey on Alcohol and Related Conditions (NESARC). Drug and alcohol dependence, 115(1-2), 120-130.

182. Lorenzetti V, et al. Adolescent cannabis use: What is the evidence for functional brain alterations? Curr Pharm Des. 2014;20(13): 2186-2198.

183. Lovejoy, J. C., Champagne, C. M., de Jonge, L., Xie, H., & Smith, S. R. (2008). Increased visceral fat and decreased energy expenditure during the menopausal transition. International Journal of Obesity, 32(6), 949-958.

184. Lowe, M. R., Butryn, M. L., & Didie, E. R. (2009). Food cravings and eating: The role of inhibitory control. Appetite, 52(3), 469-472.

185. Mairbäurl, H. (2013). Red blood cells in sports: Effects of exercise and training on oxygen supply by red blood cells. Frontiers in Physiology,4,332.doi10.3389/Phys.2013.00332

186. Marco, E. M., García-Gutiérrez, M. S., Bermúdez-Silva, F. J., Moreira, F. A., & Guimarães, F. (2012). Endocannabinoid system and psychiatry: in search of a neurobiological basis for detrimental and potential therapeutic effects. Frontiers in Behavioral Neuroscience, 6, 1-23.

187. Mark, K., Desai, A., Terplan, M. (2016). Marijuana use and pregnancy: prevalence, associated characteristics, and birth outcomes. Archives of Women's Mental Health, 19(1), 105-111.

188. Marx, J. A., Hockberger, R. S., Walls, R. M., & Adams, J. G. (Eds.). (2019). Rosen's emergency medicine: Concepts and clinical practice (9th ed.). Philadelphia, PA: Elsevier.

189. Mason, J. B., Dickstein, A., Jacques, P. F., Haggarty, P., Selhub, J., & Dallal, G. (2007). A temporal association between folic acid fortification and an increase in colorectal cancer rates may be illuminating important

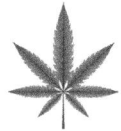

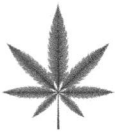

biological principles: a hypothesis. Cancer Epidemiology and Prevention Biomarkers, 16(7), 1325-1329.

190. May, P. A., Chambers, C. D., Kalberg, W. O., et al. (2018). Prevalence of Fetal Alcohol Spectrum Disorders in 4 US Communities. JAMA, 319(5), 474-482.

191. May, P. A., Chambers, C. D., Kalberg, W. O., Zellner, J., Feldman, H., Buckley, D., ... & Hoyme, H. E. (2018). Prevalence of fetal alcohol spectrum disorders in 4 US communities. JAMA, 319(5), 474-482.

192. Mayo Clinic. (2020). Alcohol withdrawal. Retrieved from https://www.mayoclinic.org/diseases-conditions/alcohol-withdrawal/symptoms-causes/syc-20369218

193. Mayo Clinic. (2020). Alcohol: What are the effects? Retrieved from https://www.mayoclinic.org/healthy-lifestyle/nutrition-and-healthy-eating/in-depth/alcohol/art-20044551

194. Mayo Clinic. (2021). Alcohol withdrawal. Retrieved from https://www.mayoclinic.org/diseases-conditions/alcohol-withdrawal/symptoms-causes/syc-20369218

195. Mayo Clinic. (2021). Antidepressants: Selecting one that's right for you. Retrieved from https://www.mayoclinic.org/diseases-conditions/depression/in-depth/antidepressants/art-20046273

196. Mayo Clinic. (2021). Chest Pain. Retrieved from https://www.mayoclinic.org/symptoms/chest-pain/basics/definition/sym-20050849

197. Mayo Clinic. (2021). Depression (major depressive disorder). Retrieved from https://www.mayoclinic.org/diseases-conditions/depression/symptoms-causes/syc-20356007

198. Mayo Clinic. (2021). Erectile Dysfunction: Diagnosis & Treatment. Retrieved from https://www.mayoclinic.org/

diaseases-conditions/erectile-dysfunction/
diagnosis-treatment/drc-20355782

199. Mayo Clinic. (2021). Hangovers. Retrieved from
https://www.mayoclinic.org/
diseases-conditions/hangovers/
symptoms-causes/syc-20373012

200. Mayo Clinic. (2021). Heart Attack.
Retrieved from https://www.mayoclinic.org/
diseases-conditions/heart-attack/
symptoms-causes/syc-20373106

201. Mazer-Amirshahi, M., & Pourmand, A. (2017).
Alternative Medicines: The Scope of Practice
and Key Principles for Emergency Physicians.
Western Journal of Emergency Medicine, 18(3),
519–526.

202. McCormack, L., & Friedland, D. J. (2002). What
do you mean, "I'm a patient"? One doctor's
plea for partnership. Annals of Internal
Medicine, 136(5), 377-381.

203. Mechoulam, R., & Parker, L. A. (2013). The
endocannabinoid system and the brain.
Annual Review of Psychology, 64, 21-47.

204. Mechoulam, R., Parker, L. A., & Gallily, R. (2002).
Cannabidiol: an overview of some
pharmacological aspects. Journal of Clinical
Pharmacology, 42(S1), 11S-19S.

205. Mehranpour, M., & Khatami, M. (2014). Gender
Differences in Hemoglobin Concentration and
Hematocrit in Elite Athletes and Different
Altitude Residents. International Journal
of Hematology-Oncology and Stem Cell
Research, 8(4), 33–36.

206. Meier MH, et al. Persistent cannabis users show
neuropsychological decline from childhood
to midlife. Proc Natl Acad Sci USA.
2012;109(40):E2657-E2664.

207. Meier, M. H., Caspi, A., Ambler, A., Harrington,
H., Houts, R., Keefe, R. S., ... & Moffitt, T. E.
(2012). Persistent cannabis users show
neuropsychological decline from childhood to
midlife. Proceedings of the National Academy

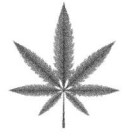

267

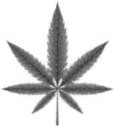

of Sciences, 109(40), E2657-E2664.

208. Meier, M. H., Caspi, A., Ambler, A., Harrington, H., Houts, R., Keefe, R. S., ... & Moffitt, T. E. (2012). Persistent cannabis users show neuropsychological decline from childhood to midlife. Proceedings of the National Academy of Sciences, 109(40), E2657-E2664.

209. Mitchell, A. A., & Cottler, L. B. (1984). Patterns of maternal drug use and the outcome of pregnancy. American Journal of Epidemiology, 119(4), 575-586. doi: 10.1093/oxfordjournals.aje.a113788

210. Morgan CJ, Curran HV. Effects of cannabidiol on schizophrenia-like symptoms in people who use cannabis. Br J Psychiatry. 2008;192(4):306-307. doi:10.1192/bjp.bp.107.046649

211. Murray, R. M., Englund, A., Abi-Dargham, A., Lewis, D. A., Di Forti, M., Davies, C., & Sherif, M. (2016). Cannabis-associated psychosis: Neural substrate and clinical impact. Neuropharmacology, 124, 89-104.

212. Murray, R. M., Quigley, H., Quattrone, D., Englund, A., & Di Forti, M. (2016). Traditional marijuana, high-potency cannabis and synthetic cannabinoids: increasing risk for psychosis. World Psychiatry, 15(3), 195-204.

213. Naderan, M., Naderan, M., Rezagholizadeh, F., & Zolfaghari, M. (2016). Vitamin D levels in tear fluid correlate with serum levels in patients with dry eye syndrome: Can vitamin D be an indicator of dry eye? Eye & Contact Lens: Science & Clinical Practice, 42(2), 124-127.

214. Naghshin, J., & Grijalva, C. G. (2017). Hemoglobin and Hematocrit. In StatPearls [Internet]. StatPearls Publishing.

215. National Academies of Sciences, Engineering, and Medicine. (2017). The health effects of cannabis and cannabinoids: The current state of evidence and recommendations for

research. The National Academies Press.

216. National Academies of Sciences, Engineering, and Medicine. (2017). The health effects of cannabis and cannabinoids: The current state of evidence and recommendations for research. Washington, DC: The National Academies Press.

217. National Academies of Sciences, Engineering, and Medicine. (2017). The health effects of cannabis and cannabinoids: The current state of evidence and recommendations for research. National Academies Press.

218. National Academies of Sciences, Engineering, and Medicine. (2017). The Health Effects of Cannabis and Cannabinoids: The Current State of Evidence and Recommendations for Re search. Washington, DC: The National Academies Press. https://doi.org/10.17226/24625

219. National Academies of Sciences, Engineering, and Medicine. (2019). Science Literacy: Concepts, Contexts, and Consequences. National Academies Press.

220. National Academy of Sciences, National Academy of Engineering, & Institute of Medicine. (1995). On being a scientist: A guide to responsible conduct in research. National Academies Press.

221. National Cancer Institute. (2021). Brain and Spinal Cord Tumors in Adults: Symptoms and Signs. Retrieved from https://www.cancer.gov/types/brain/patient/adult-brain-treatment-pdq#section/all

222. National Cancer Institute. (2022). DES (Diethylstilbestrol): Questions and Answers. Retrieved from https://www.cancer.gov/about-cancer/causes-prevention/risk/myths/des-fact-sheet

223. National Center for Complementary and Integrative Health. (2020). Complementary, alternative, or integrative

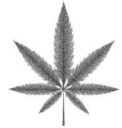

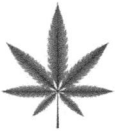

health: What's in a name? Retrieved from https://www.nccih.nih.gov/health/complementary-alternative-or-integrative-health-whats-in-a-name

224. National Center for Complementary and Integrative Health. (2021). Complementary, alternative, or integrative health: What's in a name? Retrieved from https://www.nccih.nih.gov/health/complementary-alternative-or-integrative-health-whats-in-a-name

225. National Health Service. (2021). Complementary and alternative medicine. Retrieved from https://www.nhs.uk/conditions/complementary-and-alternative-medicine/

226. National Institute of Mental Health. (2020). Autism Spectrum Disorder. Retrieved from https://www.nimh.nih.gov/health/topics/autism-spectrum-disorders-asd/index.shtml

227. National Institute of Mental Health. (2020). Depression. Retrieved from https://www.nimh.nih.gov/health/topics/depression/index.shtml

228. National Institute of Mental Health. (2021). Schizophrenia. Retrieved from https://www.nimh.nih.gov/health/topics/schizophrenia/

229. National Institute of Neurological Disorders and Stroke. (2022). Stroke: Hope Through Research. Retrieved from https://www.ninds.nih.gov/Disorders/Patient-Caregiver-Education/Hope-Through-Research/Stroke-Hope-Through-Research

230. National Institute on Alcohol Abuse and Alcoholism. (2020). Alcohol's Effects on the Body. Retrieved from https://www.niaaa.nih.gov/publications/brochures-and-fact-sheets/alcohols-effects-body

231. National Institute on Alcohol Abuse and Alcoholism. (2020). Alcohol's Effects on the Body. Retrieved from https://www.niaaa.

nih.gov/publications/brochures-and-fact-sheets/alcohols-effects-body

232. National Institute on Alcohol Abuse and Alcoholism. (2021). Alcohol Withdrawal. Retrieved from https://www.niaaa.nih.gov/alcohols-effects-health/alcohol-use-disorder/alcohol-withdrawal

233. National Institute on Alcohol Abuse and Alcoholism. (n.d.). Harmful Interactions: Mixing Alcohol with Medicines. Retrieved from https://www.niaaa.nih.gov/publications/brochures-and-fact-sheets/harmful-interactions-mixing-alcohol-with-medicines

234. National Institute on Drug Abuse. (2018). Drugs, brains, and behavior: The science of addiction. Retrieved from https://www.drugabuse.gov/publications/drugs-brains-behavior-science-addiction/introduction

235. National Institute on Drug Abuse. (2018). Understanding Drug Use and Addiction. Retrieved from https://www.drugabuse.gov/publications/drugfacts/understanding-drug-use-addiction

236. National Institute on Drug Abuse. (2018). Understanding Drug Use and Addiction. Retrieved from https://www.drugabuse.gov/publications/drugfacts/understanding-drug-use-addiction

237. National Institute on Drug Abuse. (2019). Medications to Treat Opioid Use Disorder. Retrieved from https://www.drugabuse.gov/publications/research-reports/medications-to-treat-opioid-addiction

238. National Institute on Drug Abuse. (2020). Drugs, Brains, and Behavior: The Science of Addiction. Retrieved from https://www.drugabuse.gov/publications/drugs-brains-behavior-science-addiction/drugs-brain

239. National Institute on Drug Abuse. (2020). Marijuana as medicine. Retrieved from https://

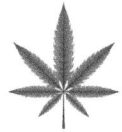

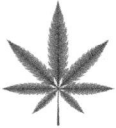

www.drugabuse.gov/publications/drugfacts/
marijuana-medicine

240. National Institute on Drug Abuse. (2020).
Marijuana as Medicine. Retrieved from https://
www.drugabuse.gov/publications/drugfacts/
marijuana-medicine

241. National Institute on Drug Abuse. (2020).
Marijuana DrugFacts. Retrieved from https://
www.drugabuse.gov/drug-topics/marijuana

242. National Institute on Drug Abuse. (2020).
Marijuana Research Report: Is Marijuana
Safe and Effective as Medicine?
Retrieved from https://www.drugabuse.gov/
publications/research-reports/marijuana/
marijuana-safe-effective-medicine

243. National Institute on Drug Abuse. (2020).
Marijuana Research Report: Is marijuana addictive?

244. National Institute on Drug Abuse. (2020).
Marijuana Research Report: What is marijuana?

245. National Institute on Drug Abuse.
(2021, June 1). Marijuana. Retrieved from
https://www.drugabuse.gov/drug-topics/marijuana

246. National Institute on Drug Abuse. (2021).
Marijuana DrugFacts. Retrieved from https://
www.drugabuse.gov/publications/
drugfacts/marijuana

247. National Institute on Drug Abuse. (2021).
Marijuana Research Report: What are
marijuana's effects?
Retrieved from https://www.drugabuse.
gov/publications/research-reports/marijuana/
what-are-marijuana-effectsAmerican
Psychological Association. (2017).
Understanding psychoanalysis. Retrieved from
https://www.apa.org/topics/psychoanalysis
American Psychoanalytic Association. (n.d.).
What is psychoanalysis? Retrieved from https://
www.apsa.org/what-is-psychoanalysis
American Psychoanalytic Association. (n.d.).
What is psychoanalysis? Retrieved from https://
www.apsa.org/what-is-psychoanalysisBersani,

G., Orlandi, V., Kotzalidis, G. D., Pancheri, P., & Valeriani, G. (2002). Cannabis and neuropsychiatry, 1: Benefits and risks. European Archives of Psychiatry and Clinical Neuroscience, 252(2), 69-74.

248. National Institute on Drug Abuse. (2021). Principles of Drug Addiction Treatment: A Research-Based Guide (Third Edition). Retrieved from https://www.drugabuse.gov/publications/principles-drug-addiction-treatment-research-based-guide-third-edition/principles-effective-treatment

249. National Institute on Drug Abuse. (2021). Substance Use and Pregnancy. Retrieved from https://www.drugabuse.gov/publications/research-reports/substance-use-in-women/substance-use-while-pregnant-breastfeeding

250. National Institute on Drug Abuse. DrugFacts: Marijuana. Accessed June 2023.

251. National Institutes of Health Office of Dietary Supplements. (2021). Folate. Retrieved from https://ods.od.nih.gov/factsheets/Folate-HealthProfessional/

252. National Research Council. (2012). A Frame work for K-12 Science Education: Practices, Crosscutting Concepts, and Core Ideas. National Academies Press.

253. Nelson, D. L., Cox, M. M. (2020). Lehninger Principles of Biochemistry. W.H. Freeman and Company.

254. Nestler, E. J. (2013). Cellular basis of memory for addiction. Dialogues in Clinical Neuroscience, 15(4), 431-443.

255. NICE. (2008). Antenatal care for uncomplicated pregnancies: Clinical guideline. Retrieved from https://www.ncbi.nlm.nih.gov/books/NBK51834/

256. Niewoehner, D. E. (1999). Pulmonary effects of marijuana inhalation. Expert Review of Respiratory Medicine, 3(4), 373-378.

257. Nisbet, M. C., & Scheufele, D. A. (2009). What's

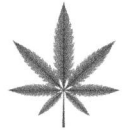

273

next for science communication? Promising directions and lingering distractions. American Journal of Botany, 96(10), 1767-1778.

258. Nugent, S. M., Morasco, B. J., O'Neil, M. E., & Freeman, M. (2017). The effects of cannabis among adults with chronic pain and an overview of general harms: a systematic review. Annals of Internal Medicine, 167(5), 319-331.

259. Nutbeam, D. (2000). Health literacy as a public health goal: a challenge for contemporary health education and communication strategies into the 21st century. Health Promotion International, 15(3), 259-267. doi: 10.1093/heapro/15.3.259

260. Nutt, D., King, L. A., & Phillips, L. D. (2010). Drug harms in the UK: a multicriteria decision analysis. The Lancet, 376(9752), 1558-1565.

261. Ockene, I. S., Miller, N. H., & Cigarette Smoking Cessation Intervention Trial Research Group. (2003). Cigarette smoking, cardiovascular disease, and stroke: a statement for healthcare professionals from the American Heart Association. Circulation, 102(23), 3046-3053.

262. Office of Dietary Supplements - National Institutes of Health. (2021). Vitamin B12. Retrieved from https://ods.od.nih.gov/factsheets/VitaminB12-HealthProfessional/

263. Omerov, P., Steineck, G., Runeson, B., & Christensson, A. C. (2019). The individual's important role in the therapeutic alliance during cancer treatment: a longitudinal study reviewing alliance, individual distress, and anxiety in women with breast cancer. Journal of psychosocial oncology, 37(3), 305-319.

264. Ong, L. M., de Haes, J. C., Hoos, A. M., & Lammes, F. B. (1995). Doctor-patient communication: a review of the literature. Social science & medicine, 40(7), 903-918.

265. Pearl, J. (2009). Causality: Models, reasoning, and inference. Cambridge University Press.

266. Pertwee RG. Cannabinoid pharmacology: the

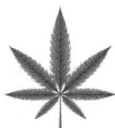

274

first 66 years. Br J Pharmacol. 2006;147 Suppl 1(Suppl 1):S163-S171. doi:10.1038/sj. bj.0706406

267. Pertwee, R. G. (2008). The diverse CB1 and CB2 receptor pharmacology of three plant cannabinoids: Δ9-tetrahydrocannabinol, cannabidiol and Δ9-tetrahydrocannabivarin. British Journal of Pharmacology, 153(2), 199-215. doi: 10.1038/sj. bj.0707442

268. Pi-Sunyer, F. X. (2009). The medical risks of obesity. Postgraduate Medicine, 121(6), 21-33.

269. Pichini, S., Pacifici, R., & Busardò, F. P. (2018). Pharmacokinetic, metabolic, and analytical aspects of synthetic cannabinoids. Handbook of Experimental Pharmacology, 252, 95-107.

270. Pirmohamed, M. (2016). Drug-grapefruit juice interactions: two mechanisms are clear but individual responses vary. British Journal of Clinical Pharmacology, 81(5), 918-920.

271. Pistis, M., & Melis, M. (2010). From surface to nuclear receptors: the endocannabinoid family extends its assets. Current Medicinal Chemistry, 17(14), 1450-1467.

272. Ponganis, P. J. (2011). Diving physiology of marine mammals and seabirds. Cambridge University Press.

273. Quigley, H. A., & Broman, A. T. (2006). The number of people with glaucoma worldwide in 2010 and 2020. British Journal of Ophthalmology, 90(3), 262-267.

274. Ramaekers, J. G., Berghaus, G., van Laar, M., & Drummer, O. H. (2004). Dose related risk of motor vehicle crashes after cannabis use. Drug and Alcohol Dependence, 73(2), 109-119.

275. Rang, H. P., Dale, M. M., Ritter, J. M., & Flower, R. J. (2020). Rang & Dale's Pharmacology (9th ed.). Elsevier.

276. Ranganathan, M., & D'Souza, D. C. (2006). The acute effects of cannabinoids on memory in humans: a review. Psychopharmacology, 188(4), 425-444.

277. Ravi, D., Ghasemiesfe, M., Korenstein, D.,

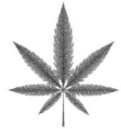

275

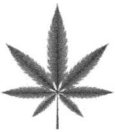

Cascino, T., & Keyhani, S. (2017). Associations between marijuana use and cardiovascular risk factors and outcomes: a systematic review. Annals of Internal Medicine, 167(5), 319-331.

278. Rendic, S., & Guengerich, F. P. (2015). Drug–drug interactions for UDP-glucuronosyl transferase substrates: a pharmacokinetic explanation for typically observed low exposure (AUCi/AUC) ratios. Drug Metabolism and Disposition, 43(1), 98-100.

279. Reynolds, E. H. (2006). Benefits and risks of folic acid to the nervous system. Journal of Neurology, Neurosurgery & Psychiatry, 77(8), 1097-1099.

280. Ridgway, S. H., & Harrison, R. J. (2001). Handbook of marine mammals: The second book of dolphins and the porpoises. Academic Press.

281. Riley, E. P., & Infante, M. A. (2018). Warren, W. K. Fetal Alcohol Spectrum Disorders: An Overview. Neuropsychology Review, 28(2), 94-107.

282. Riley, E. P., Infante, M. A., & Warren, K. R. (2011). Fetal alcohol spectrum disorders: an overview. Neuropsychology Review, 21(2), 73-80.

283. Röhrich, J., Schimmel, I., Zörntlein, S., et al. (2010). Concentrations of Δ9-tetrahydrocannabinol and 11-nor-9-carboxytetrahydrocannabinol in blood and urine after passive exposure to Cannabis smoke in a coffee shop. Journal of Analytical Toxicology, 34(4), 196-203.

284. Rollnick, S., Miller, W. R., & Butler, C. (2008). Motivational interviewing in health care: Helping patients change behavior. Guilford Press.

285. Romano, E., & Voas, R. B. (2011). Drug and alcohol involvement in four types of fatal crashes. Journal of Studies on Alcohol and Drugs, 72(4), 567-576.

286. Rothman, K. J., Greenland, S., & Lash,

T. L. (2008). Modern epidemiology. Lippincott Williams & Wilkins.

287. Russo EB. Cannabinoids in the management of difficult to treat pain. Therapeutics and Clinical Risk Management. 2008 Feb;4(1):245-59.

288. Russo EB. Cannabinoids in the management of difficult-to-treat pain. Ther Clin Risk Manag. 2008;4(1):245-259. doi:10.2147/tcrm.s1928

289. Russo EB. Cannabinoids in the management of difficult-to-treat pain. Ther Clin Risk Manag. 2008;4(1):245-259. doi:10.2147/tcrm.s1928

290. Russo EB. Cannabis and Cannabinoids: Pharmacology, Toxicology, and Therapeutic Potential. Routledge, 2013.

291. Russo, E. B. (2008). Cannabinoids in the management of difficult-to-treat pain. Therapeutics and Clinical Risk Management, 4(1), 245-259. doi: 10.2147/TCRM.S1928

292. Ryan, S. A., Ammerman, S. D., O'Connor, M. E., & Committee on Substance Use and Prevention. (2018). Marijuana use during pregnancy and breastfeeding: implications for neonatal and childhood outcomes. Pediatrics, 142(3), e20181889.

293. Sacchetti, M., Lambiase, A., & Mantelli, F. (2013). Focus on the role of vitamins in the prevention and treatment of ocular surface diseases. International Journal of Molecular Sciences, 14(5), 18325-18341.

294. Salo, D. C., & Pacifici, G. M. (2007). Oxygen and carbon dioxide transport. In M. G. Levitzky (Ed.), Pulmonary physiology (7th ed., pp. 33-43). McGraw-Hill Medical.

295. Schauer, G. L., King, B. A., Bunnell, R. E., Promoff, G., & McAfee, T. A. (2016). Toking, Vaping, and Eating for Health or Fun: Marijuana Use Patterns in Adults, US, 2014. American Journal of Preventive Medicine, 50(1), 1-8.

296. Schoeler, T., Bhattacharyya, S., & Stefanis, N. C.

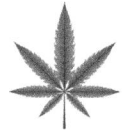

277

(2013). The effect of cannabis use on memory function: an update. Substance Abuse and Rehabilitation, 4, 11-27.

297. Schuckit, M. A. (2014). Alcohol-use disorders. The Lancet, 383(9919), 988-998.

298. Schuckit, M. A. (2016). Drug and alcohol abuse: A clinical guide to diagnosis and treatment. Springer.

299. Schuckit, M. A. (2016). Drug and alcohol abuse: A clinical guide to diagnosis and treatment. Springer.

300. Schuel, H., Burkman, L. J., Lippes, J., Crickard, K., Mahony, M. C., Giuffrida, A., ... & Evans, T. (2002). Evidence that anandamide-signaling regulates human sperm functions required for fertilization. Molecular Reproduction and Development: Incorporating Gamete Research, 63(3), 376-387.

301. Schuster, R. M., Crane, N. A., Mermelstein, R. J., & Gonzalez, R. (2012). The influence of inhibitory control and episodic memory on the risky sexual behavior of young adult cannabis users. Journal of the International Neuropsychological Society, 18(5), 827-833.

302. Schwope, D. M., Bosker, W. M., Ramaekers, J. G., Gorelick, D. A., Huestis, M. A. (2012). Psychomotor performance, subjective and physiological effects, and whole blood Δ9-tetrahydrocannabinol concentrations in heavy, chronic cannabis smokers following acute smoked cannabis. J Analytical Toxicology, 36(6), 405–412.

303. Scott, J. C., Slomiak, S. T., Jones, J. D., Rosen, A. F., Moore, T. M., & Gur, R. C. (2018). Association of cannabis with cognitive functioning in adolescents and young adults: A systematic review and meta-analysis. JAMA Psychiatry, 75(6), 585-595.

304. Scott, J. C., Slomiak, S. T., Jones, J. D., Rosen, A. F., Moore, T. M., & Gur, R. C. (2018). Association of cannabis with cognitive

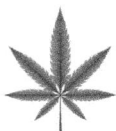

functioning in adolescents and young adults: a systematic review and meta-analysis. JAMA Psychiatry, 75(6), 585-595

305. Selhub, J. (2006). Homocysteine metabolism. Annual Review of Nutrition, 26, 209-235.

306. Sexton, B. F., Tunbridge, R. J., Jackson, P. G., & Shanahan, M. (2019). Cannabis, alcohol and fatal road accidents. Forensic Science International, 298, 161-166.

307. Shields, P. G., & Mello, N. K. (2020). Cannabis smoking: Effects on the lung. In Principles of Addiction: Comprehensive Addictive Behaviors and Disorders (Vol. 1, pp. 440-453). Academic Press.

308. Shiffman, S. (2009). Tobacco "chippers" – Individual differences in tobacco dependence. Psychopharmacology, 207(3), 365-367.

309. Sigmon, S. C., Herning, R. I., Better, W., Cadet, J. L., & Griffiths, R. R. (2009). Caffeine withdrawal, acute effects, tolerance, and absence of net beneficial effects of chronic administration: Cerebral blood flow velocity, quantitative EEG, and subjective effects. Psychopharmacology, 204(4), 573-585.

310. Silverthorn, D. U. (2018). Human Physiology: An Integrated Approach (8th ed.). Pearson.

311. Sirdifield, C., & Chipchase, S. Y. (2013). Evidence-based medicine: a concise guide for clinicians. International Journal of Clinical Practice, 67(9), 847-850.

312. Smith, R. (2011). Why do patients fail to comply with treatment regimens? British Journal of General Practice, 61(588), 652-654.

313. Stewart, M., Brown, J. B., Donner, A., McWhinney, I. R., Oates, J., Weston, W. W., & Jordan, J. (2000). The impact of patient-centered care on outcomes. Journal of Family Practice, 49(9), 796-804.

314. Stout, S. M., & Cimino, N. M. (2014). Exogenous cannabinoids as substrates, inhibitors, and inducers of human drug metabolizing enzymes:

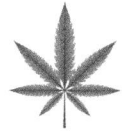

a systematic review. Drug Metabolism Reviews, 46(1), 86-95.

315. Stout, S. M., Cimino, N. M., & Satin, L. S. (2019). Cannabis use and its implications in the world of medicine: A comprehensive review. Forensic Science and Medicine, 5(2), 105-118.

316. Straiker, A., Stella, N., Piomelli, D., Mackie, K., & Karten, H. J. (1999). Cannabinoid CB1 receptors and ligands in vertebrate retina: Localization and function of an endogenous signaling system. Proceedings of the National Academy of Sciences, 96(25), 14565-14570.

317. Straus, S. E., & Sackett, D. L. (2018). Using research findings in clinical practice. BMJ, 358, j3990.

318. Substance Abuse and Mental Health Services Administration. (2019). Key substance use and mental health indicators in the United States: Results from the 2018 National Survey on Drug Use and Health.

319. Substance Abuse and Mental Health Services Administration. (2020). Methadone. Retrieved from https://www.samhsa.gov/medication-assisted-treatment/treatment/methadone

320. Sullivan, J. T., & Sykora, K. (1989). The alcohol withdrawal syndrome. JAMA, 261(24), 3615-3619.

321. Tarnawski, A. (2011). Cellular and molecular mechanisms of gastrointestinal ulcer healing. Digestive Diseases and Sciences, 56(8), 2019-2026. doi: 10.1007/s10620-011-1720-1

322. Tashkin, D. P. (2013). Effects of marijuana smoking on the lung. Annals of the American Thoracic Society, 10(3), 239-247.

323. Taylor H, Freeman TP, Munafo MR, et al. Meta-analysis of the association between cannabis use and risk of psychosis. Schizophrenia Bulletin. 2020 Jan;46(1):110-7.

324. Taylor, D. R., Poulton, R., Moffitt, T. E., Ramankutty, P., & Sears, M. R. (2000). The respiratory effects of cannabis

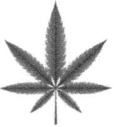

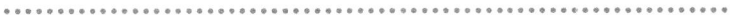

dependence in young adults.
Addiction, 95(11), 1669-1677.

325. Taylor, L. E., Swerdfeger, A. L., & Eslick, G. D. (2014). Vaccines are not associated with autism: an evidence-based meta-analysis of case-control and cohort studies. Vaccine, 32(29), 3623-3629.

326. Thapa D, Cairns EA, Suleymanova N, Toguri JT, Cloutier CJ. The Cannabinoids Δ8THC, CBD, and HU-308 Act via Distinct Receptors to Reduce Corneal Pain and Inflammation. Cannabis Cannabinoid Res. 2018;3(1):11-20. doi:10.1089/can.2017.0041

327. The American Academy of Ophthalmology. (2021). Angle-closure glaucoma. Retrieved from https://www.aao.org/eye-health/diseases/angle-closure-glaucoma

328. The American Academy of Ophthalmology. (2021). Primary open-angle glaucoma. Retrieved from https://www.aao.org/eye-health/diseases/primary-open-angle-glaucoma-2

329. The American Glaucoma Society. (2021). Marijuana and glaucoma. Retrieved from https://www.americanglaucomasociety.net/marijuana-and-glaucoma

330. Thomas, G., Kloner, R. A., & Rezkalla, S. (2014). Adverse cardiovascular, cerebrovascular, and peripheral vascular effects of marijuana inhalation: what cardiologists need to know. American Journal of Cardiology, 113(1), 187-190.

331. Tomida, I., Azuara-Blanco, A., House, H., Flint, M., Pertwee, R. G., & Robson, P. J. (2006). Effect of Sublingual Application of Cannabinoids on Intraocular Pressure: A Pilot Study. Journal of Glaucoma, 15(5), 349-353.

332. Tomida, I., Azuara-Blanco, A., House, H., Flint, M., Pertwee, R. G., & Robson, P. J. (2006). Effect of sublingual application of cannabinoids on

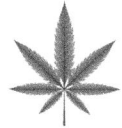

281

intraocular pressure: A pilot study. Journal of Glaucoma, 15(5), 349-353.

333. Tortora, G. J., Derrickson, B. H. (2017). Principles of Anatomy and Physiology (15th ed.). John Wiley & Sons.

334. U.S. Department of Health and Human Services. (2014). The Health Consequences of Smoking—50 Years of Progress: A Report of the Surgeon General. Retrieved from https://www.ncbi.nlm.nih.gov/books/NBK179276/

335. United States Federal Trade Commission. (2019). Health claims in advertising. Retrieved from https://www.ftc.gov/system/files/documents/plain-language/bus41-health-claims-advertising.pdf

336. US Preventive Services Task Force. (2018). Folic acid supplementation for the prevention of neural tube defects: US Preventive Services Task Force recommendation statement. JAMA, 319(2), 151-157.

337. Valko, M., et al. (2007). Free radicals and anti oxidants in normal physiological functions and human disease. The International Journal of Biochemistry & Cell Biology, 39(1), 44-84.

338. Vandenbroucke, J. P. (2008). Observational research, randomised trials, and two views of medical science. PLoS Medicine, 5(3), e67.

339. Vidyasagar, A., & Wilson, N. A. (2018). Epithelial structure and function in the pathogenesis of asthma. Translational Research, 201, 1-11. doi: 10.1016/j.trsl.2018.07.006

340. Volkow ND, et al. Adverse Health Effects of Marijuana Use. N Engl J Med. 2014;370(23):2219-2227. doi:10.1056/NEJMra1402309

341. Volkow ND, et al. Effects of cannabis use on human behaviour, including cognition, motivation, and psychosis: A review. JAMA Psychiatry. 2016;73(3):292-297.

342. Volkow ND, Swanson JM, Evins AE, et al. Effects of Cannabis Use on Human Behavior, Including

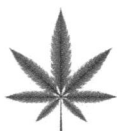

Cognition, Motivation, and Psychosis: A Review. JAMA Psychiatry. 2016 Jun;73(3):292-7.

343. Volkow ND, Swanson JM, Evins AE, et al. Effects of cannabis use on human behaviour, including cognition, motivation, and psychosis: a review. JAMA Psychiatry. 2016;73(3):292-297. doi:10.1001/jamapsychiatry.2015.3278

344. Volkow, N. D., & McLellan, A. T. (2016). Opioid abuse in chronic pain—Misconceptions and mitigation strategies. New England Journal of Medicine, 374(13), 1253-1263.

345. Volkow, N. D., & Morales, M. (2015). The Brain on Drugs: From Reward to Addiction. Cell, 162(4), 712-725.

346. Volkow, N. D., Baler, R. D., Compton, W. M., & Weiss, S. R. (2014). Adverse health effects of marijuana use. New England Journal of Medicine, 370(23), 2219-2227.

347. Volkow, N. D., Compton, W. M., & Weiss, S. R. (2014). Adverse health effects of marijuana use. New England Journal of Medicine, 371(9), 879-879.

348. Volkow, N. D., et al. (2014). Adverse health effects of marijuana use. New England Journal of Medicine, 370(23), 2219-2227.

349. Volkow, N. D., Han, B., Compton, W. M., McCance-Katz, E. F. (2019). Self-reported medical and nonmedical cannabis use among pregnant women in the United States. JAMA, 322(2), 167-169.

350. Volkow, N. D., Han, B., Compton, W. M., McCance-Katz, E. F., & Substance Abuse and Mental Health Services Administration. (2019). Self-reported Medical and Nonmedical Cannabis Use Among Pregnant Women in the United States. JAMA: Journal of the American Medical Association, 322(2), 167-169. doi:10.1001/jama.2019.7982

351. Wang T, Collet JP, Shapiro S, et al. Adverse effects of medical cannabinoids: a systematic

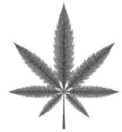

review. CMAJ. 2008;178(13):1669-1678. doi:10.1503/cmaj.071178

352. Wartman, S. A., & Morlock, L. L. (2011). The impact of the internet on health outcomes. Mount Sinai Journal of Medicine: A Journal of Translational and Personalized Medicine, 78(6), 843-851.

353. Weinreb, R. N., Aung, T., & Medeiros, F. A. (2014). The pathophysiology and treatment of glaucoma: A review. JAMA, 311(18), 1901-1911.

354. Weinreb, R. N., Aung, T., & Medeiros, F. A. (2014). The pathophysiology and treatment of glaucoma: A review. JAMA, 311(18), 1901-1911.

355. West, J. B. (2016). Respiratory physiology: the essentials. Wolters Kluwer.

356. Whiting, P. F., et al. (2015). Cannabinoids for medical use: A systematic review and meta-analysis. JAMA, 313(24), 2456-2473.

357. Whiting, P. F., Wolff, R. F., Deshpande, S., Di Nisio, M., Duffy, S., Hernandez, A. V., ... & Kleijnen, J. (2015). Cannabinoids for medical use: A systematic review and meta-analysis. JAMA, 313(24), 2456-2473.

358. Widmaier, E. P., et al. (2019). Vander's Human Physiology: The Mechanisms of Body Function (15th ed.). McGraw-Hill Education.

359. Wilkinson, G. R. (2005). Drug metabolism and variability among patients in drug response. New England Journal of Medicine, 352(21), 2211-2221.

360. World Health Organization. (2018). Cannabis: WHO position paper. Retrieved from https://www.who.int/medicines/access/controlled-substances/5.2_Cannabis_review.pdf

361. World Health Organization. (2020). Tobacco and heart disease. Retrieved from https://www.who.int/news-room/fact-sheets/detail/tobacco

362. World Health Organization. (2021). Alcohol. Retrieved from https://www.who.int/news-room/fact-sheets/detail/alcohol

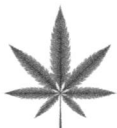

363. World Health Organization. (2021). HIV/AIDS. Retrieved from https://www.who.int/health-topics/hiv-aids#tab=tab_1

364. World Health Organization. (2021). Tobacco. Retrieved from https://www.who.int/news-room/fact-sheets/detail/tobacco

365. Wu, G., et al. (2004). Ascorbic Acid in Bronchoalveolar Lavage Fluid of Patients with Asthma. American Journal of Respiratory and Critical Care Medicine, 170(8), 842-847.

366. Yawn, B. P., Wollan, P. C., & Weingarten, T. N. (2009). Hereditary angioedema: A primer for physicians. Mayo Clinic Proceedings, 84(4), 349-357. doi: 10.1016/S0025-6196(11)60555-5

367. Yeh, E. T., & Bickford, C. L. (2009). Cardiovascular complications of cancer therapy: incidence, pathogenesis, diagnosis, and management. Journal of the American College of Cardiology, 53(24), 2231-2247.

368. Yetley, E. A. (2007). Multivitamin and multimineral dietary supplements: definitions, characterization, bioavailability, and drug interactions. The American Journal of Clinical Nutrition, 85(1), 269S-276S.

369. Zanger, U. M., & Schwab, M. (2013). Cytochrome P450 enzymes in drug metabolism: Regulation of gene expression, enzyme activities, and impact of genetic variation. Pharmacology & Therapeutics, 138(1), 103-141.

370. Zanger, U. M., & Schwab, M. (2013). Cytochrome P450 enzymes in drug metabolism: Regulation, genetic variation and clinical relevance. Drug Metabolism and Drug Interactions, 28(1), 1-6.

371. Zanger, U. M., & Schwab, M. (2013). Cytochrome P450 enzymes in drug metabolism: regulation of gene expression, enzyme activities, and impact of genetic variation. Pharmacology & Therapeutics, 138(1), 103-141.

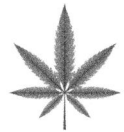

372. Zanini, C., Rasero, L., Tamburini, M., & Frova, L. (2016). Appropriateness of the patients' demand for emergency department care: an observational study. BMC Emergency Medicine, 16(1), 30.

373. Zerbo, O., Qian, Y., Yoshida, C., Grether, J. K., Van de Water, J., & Croen, L. A. (2019). Maternal infection during pregnancy and autism spectrum disorders. Journal of Autism and Developmental Disorders, 49(3), 1076-1085.

374. Zikmund-Fisher, B. J., & Fagerlin, A. (2018). Uptake and use of actionable information from health risk appraisals. In Shared Decision Making in Health Care (pp. 195-206). Oxford University Press.

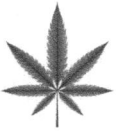

286

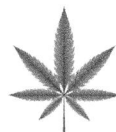

287

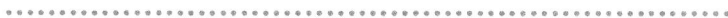

www.ingramcontent.com/pod-product-compliance
Lightning Source LLC
Chambersburg PA
CBHW062120020426
42335CB00013B/1036